Cancer Cure Is Found

Laetrile is the answer

CANCER CURE IS FOUND
Laetrile is the answer

During 1950, a biochemist Dr. Ernest T. Krebs Jr., isolated a new vitamin from bitter apricot kernel that he called 'B-17' or 'Laetrile'. He conducted further lab animal and culture experiments to conclude that laetrile would be effective in the treatment of cancer. He proposed that cancer was caused by a deficiency of Vitamin B 17 (Laetrile, Amygdaline). Laetrile is a concentrated and purified form of vitamin B17. After a lot of research, he had finally developed a specific protocol to treat cancer. Laetrile Therapy combines Laetrile with nutritional supplements and a healthy diet to create a potent treatment that fights cancer cells while helping to strengthen the body's immune system.

Vitamin B-17, which is present in several different foods, consists of a locked substance which comprises two units glucose, one unit benzaldehyde and one unit cyanide. When B17 comes in contact with a cancer cell it is unlocked by a hormone found only in the cancer cell, and becomes a lethal chemical bomb which destroys the cancer cell. Healthy cells do not cause breakdown of B17. Cancer is unknown to people living in areas with food products rich in B-17, and the population lives to a remarkably high age. Apparently nature has provided us with an ingenious defense against cancer, and it is an ordinary nutrient in our food. These are, amongst others nuts, seeds, vegetables, and in particular apricot kernels.

At present, patients listen or read a lot about Laetrile treatment, but usually they don't get precise and to the point information about what are the exact components of this protocol, where to get Laetrile injections and supplements, what to take, what not to take, what are the doses, how long to take the treatment, what diet they have to follow, etc. In this book, I have explained the protocol in detail proposed by Dr. Krebs. I have given every minute detail about Laetrile, other nutritional supplements and diet in this book. After reading this book patients can buy Laetrile injections, tablets and other nutritional supplements from the reliable sources (given in the book) and conduct the treatment under the supervision of their family doctor. Dr. Philip E. Binzel was personally trained by Dr. Ernest T Kreb Jr. about everything of this treatment. Dr. Binzel had been using Laetrile therapy in the treatment of cancer patients since the mid 1970s. His record of success was astounding. Testimonies of his patients are also included in this book.

Dr. Om Verma

~~**~~

Copyright © 2014 by Dr. O.P.Verma

All rights reserved

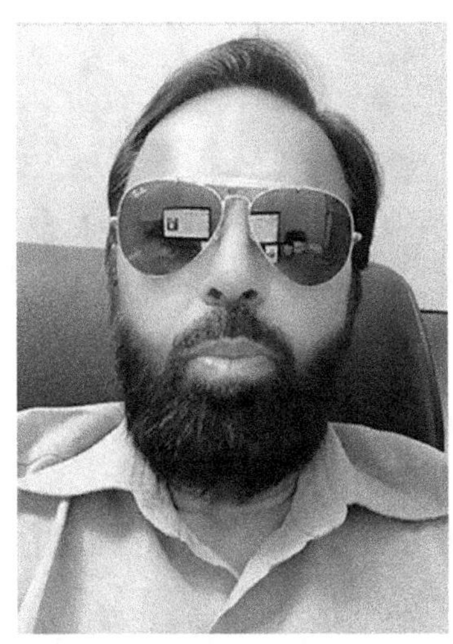

Written by
Dr. O.P.Verma
M.B.B.S., M.R.S.H. (London)
President, Flax Awareness Society
7-B-43, Mahaveer Nagar III, Kota (Raj.)
http://Flaxindia.blogspot.in
http://budwig.in
+919460816360

Table Of Content

Discovery of Laetrile

During 1950, after many years of research, a dedicated biochemist Dr. Ernst T. Krebs Jr., isolated a new substance from bitter apricot kernel that he called 'B-17'. He conducted further lab animal and culture experiments to conclude that laetrile would be effective in the treatment of cancer. He developed the compound into the injectable chemical known as "Laetrile or B17." As the years rolled by, thousands became convinced that Krebs had finally found the treatment for all cancers. He proposed that cancer was caused by a deficiency of Vitamin B 17 (Laetrile, Amygdaline).

Nitriloside is a beta-cyanophoric glycosides, a large group of water-soluble, sugar-containing compounds found in a number of plants. Amygdalin is one of the most common nitrilosides. Laetrile is a partly man-made molecule and shares only part of the amygdalin structure. Both Laetrile and amygdalin have been promoted as "Vitamin B-17".

Laetrile stands for laevo-rotatory mandelonitrile beta-diglucoside. The "laevo" part references a purified form of B-17 that turns polarized light in a left-turning direction. Dr. Krebs Jr. discovered that only this left-turning form of Laetrile was effective against cancer. "Laetrile" (with a capital "L") usually refers to the Krebses' original product, whose purification process was patented by them; "laetrile" (with a lower case "l") refers to the commercial form of amygdalin which is most likely a mixture of the left and right-turning forms, which the Krebses believed to be much less effective as a therapy for cancer. Natural amygdalin with the right turning configuration can be racemized to the unnatural form, neoamygdaline, during inexperienced extraction, bad packing or storage. So it's important to check the purity of your Laetrile.

Sources of Vitamin B-17

There are more than 1200 plants that contain nitriloside or laetrile (Vitamin B 17). Bitter Apricot seeds have the highest content of B-17 on earth. Here are some of the major foods that contain this amazing cancer fighting Laetrile:

1. Seeds of Fruits or Kernels: Seeds of bitter apricot, cherry, apple, peach, plum, pear & prune contain good amounts of laetrile.

2. Nuts: Macadamia, Bitter Almond and Walnuts.

3. Beans: Burma, Broad (Vicia faba), lentils (sprouted), green bean (sprouted), lima, Scarlet runner, Rangoon.

4. Berries: Nearly all wild berries- Chokeberry, Blackberry, Christmas berry, Elderberry, Raspberry, Cranberry, Strawberry.

5. Grasses: Acacia, Aquatic, Alfa alfa (sprouted), Milkweed, Sudan, Minus, white dover, wheat grass.

6. Seeds: Flax, Chia, Sesame.

How Vitamin B-17 works (A tale of two enzymes)

Laetrile, commonly known as Vitamin B-17 or Amygdalin, contains two units of Sugar, one of Benzaldehyde and one of Cyanide, all tightly locked within it. Everyone knows that cyanide can be highly toxic and even fatal if taken in sufficient quantity. However, as it is in locked state is completely inert and absolutely has no effect on living tissue. There is only one substance that can unlock this molecule and release the cyanide. That substance is an enzyme called beta-glucocidase, which we shall call the unlocking enzyme. When B-17 comes in contact with this enzyme, not only the cyanide is released but also Benzaldehyde which is highly toxic by itself. In fact, these two working together are at least 100 times more poisonous to cancer cell than either of them separately. The unlocking enzyme is not found to any dangerous degree anywhere in the body except at the cancer cell where it is present in great quantity. The result is that Vitamin B-17 is unlocked at the cancer cells becomes poisonous to the cancer cells and only to the cancer cells.

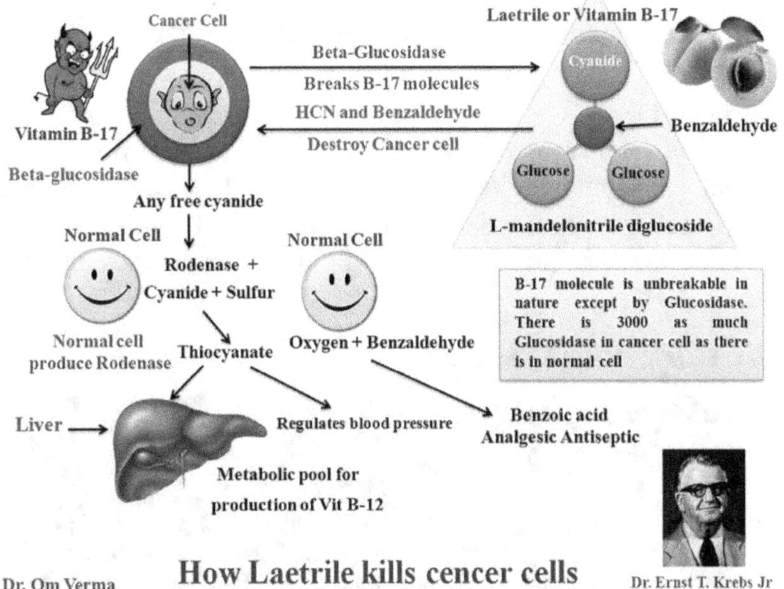

How Laetrile kills cencer cells

There is another important enzyme called Rodanese, which we shall identify as protecting enzyme. The reason is that it has the ability to neutralize cyanide by converting it instantly into the byproducts (thiocyanate) that actually are beneficial and essential for health. This enzyme also oxidizes the Benzaldehyde to produce Benzoic Acid which is natural pain killer. This enzyme is found in great quantities in every part of the body except the cancer cells which consequently is not protected. Here then is a biochemical process that destroys cancer cells while at the same time nourishing and sustaining non-cancerous cells. It is intricate and perfect mechanism of nature that simply couldn't be accidental.

It has Cyanide still Is it really safe?

I should also clarify the misconception that laetrile contains highly lethal chemical cyanide. But it does contain cyanide ion (-CN), not the chemical cyanide. When laetrile is metabolized in the body it is converted to thiocyanate, a relatively non-toxic product that has inhibitory effect against cancer (Contreras, 1982). Vitamin B-12 (Cyanocobalamin) also contain cyanide ion, but that is absolutely safe and essential for our body.

To prove that it was not toxic to humans he injected it into his own arm. As he predicted, there were no harmful or distressing side effects. The Laetrile had no harmful effect on normal cells but was deadly to cancer cells. Dr. Ernst Krebs stated that we need at least a minimum of 100 mg of B-17 or around 10 bitter apricot seeds to almost guarantee a cancer free life.

The story of the Hunza

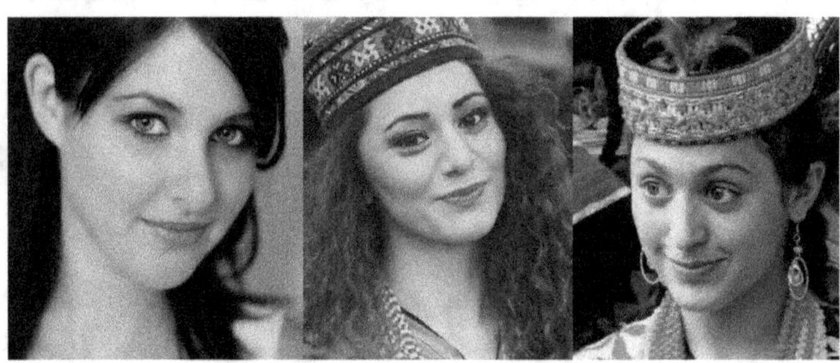

In the remote recesses of the Himalaya Mountains, between West Pakistan, India, and China, there is a tiny kingdom called Hunza. These people are known world over for their amazing longevity and good health. It is not uncommon for Hunzakuts to live beyond a hundred years, and some even to a hundred and twenty or more. Visiting medical teams from the outside world have reported that they found no cancer in Hunza. Although presently accepted science is unable to explain why these people should have been free of cancer, it is interesting to note that the traditional Hunza diet contains over two-hundred times more nitriloside than the average American diet.

In fact, in that land where there was no such thing as money; a man's wealth was measured by the number of apricot trees he owned. And the most prized of all foods was considered to be the apricot seed. One of the first medical teams to gain access to the remote kingdom of Hunza was headed by the world-renowned British surgeon and physician Dr. Robert McCarrison.

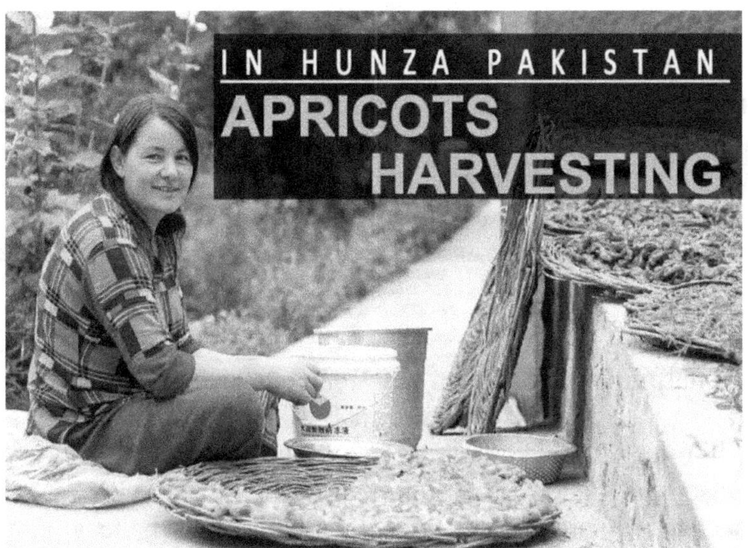

The women of Hunza are renowned for their strikingly smooth skin even into advanced age. Generally, their faces appear fifteen to twenty years younger than their counterparts in other areas of the world. They claim that their secret is merely the apricot oil which they apply to their skins almost daily. It is not surprising, therefore, to learn that westernized man is victimized by the chronic metabolic disease of cancer while his counterpart in Hunza is not. And lest anyone suspect that this difference is due to hereditary factors, it is important to know that when the Hunzakuts leave their secluded land and adopt the menus of other countries, they soon succumb to the same diseases and infirmities—including cancer—as the rest of mankind.

The Eskimos are another people that have been observed by medical teams for many decades and found to be totally free of cancer. In Vilhjalmur Stefanson's book, Cancer: Disease of

Civilization? An Anthropological and Historical Study,(2) it is revealed that the traditional Eskimo diet is amazingly rich in nitrilosides that come from the residue of the meat of caribou and other grazing animals, and also from the salmon berry which grows abundantly in the Arctic areas.

Another Eskimo delicacy is a green salad made out of the stomach contents of caribou and reindeer which are full of fresh tundra grasses. Among these grasses, Arrow grass (Triglochin Maritima) is very common. Studies made by the U.S. Department of Agriculture have shown that Arrow grass is probably richer in nitriloside content than any other grass. (World Without Cancer)

Vitamin B-15

Vitamin B-15 has been mentioned as an important auxiliary therapy to vitamin B-17. Vitamin B-15 is called pangamic acid. Pan implies everywhere and gami means seed. It was so named because it is found in small amounts almost everywhere on earth in seeds and usually with the other members of the vitamin-B complex. Like Vitamin B-17, it was also discovered by Dr. E.T. Krebs, while exploring the chemical properties of bitter apricot kernels in 1952. It was an unexpected bonus or by-product of the search for vitamin B-17. It was part of vitamin B group up to 1970.

The best way to understand the effect of vitamin B-15 is to think of it as instant oxygen. It increases the oxygen efficiency of the entire body and aids in the detoxification of waste products. Since cancer cells do not thrive in the presence of oxygen but depend rather on fermentation of glucose, it is probable that B-15, indirectly, is an enemy of cancer.

It has been reported that the Russian athletes have been given heavy doses of B-15 during their participation at the Olympics. If this is true, there is good reason for it. Experiments have shown that this substance, although just a natural food factor, greatly increases physical strength and stamina (Dr Robert E. Willner M.D., 1993).

B-15 has also been used to treat fatigue, general stress, headaches, asthma, autism, high serum cholesterol, atherosclerosis, hypertension, shortness of breath, angina, premature aging, insomnia, rheumatism, musculoskeletal chest pain and alcohol problems, possibly reducing the craving and hang over.

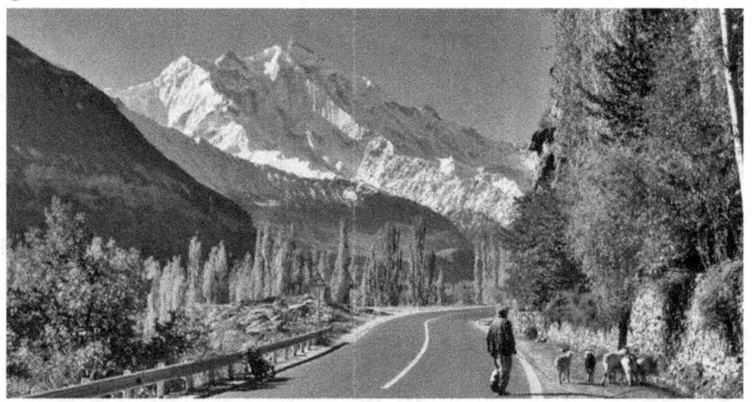

Science and Politics of Laetrile

The pharmaceutical companies, unable to patent or claim exclusive rights to the Laetrile, launched a propaganda attack against B-17, despite the fact that hard proof of its efficiency in controlling all forms of cancer surrounds us in overwhelming abundance. Why has orthodox medicine waged war against this non-profit non-drug approach? G. Edward Griffin, author of the book "World Without Cancer" states that the answer is to be found not in science, but in politics of cancer, and is based upon the hidden economic and power agenda of those who dominate the medical establishment.

In the U.S. the FDA has tried to use unfair tactics, not law, to denounce vitamin B-17 in early seventies. Vitamin B-17, or Laetrile Therapy still used in Mexico, Italy, Israel, Switzerland, Germany, Russia, Japan and many other countries.

Although it was not approved for treatment, doctors like John A. Richardson M.D. began using it "illegally" to treat patients at his clinic in San Francisco, and it was working remarkably better than orthodox treatments. His success with laetrile is well documented in his book "Laetrile Case Histories".

Early in 1974, the California medical board brought formal charges against Stewart M. Jones, M.D., for using Laetrile in the treatment of cancer patients. It was learned later, however, that Dr. Julius Levine, one of the members of that board, himself had been using Laetrile in the treatment of his own cancer. When Dr. Jones' case came up for review, the political pressures were so great that Dr. Levine felt compelled to resign from his post rather than come out openly in support of Dr. Jones and his patients. All this happened in a democratic country whose national symbol is the Statue of Liberty.

Dr. Dean Burk, the former head of the Cytochemistry Department of the National Cancer Institute, and one of the co-founders of this famous American medical institution, had worked on Vitamin B-17 personally. He described, "When we added laetrile to a cancer culture under the microscope, we observed the cancer cells dying off like flies. What a scene! I saw thousand dreams of "World Without 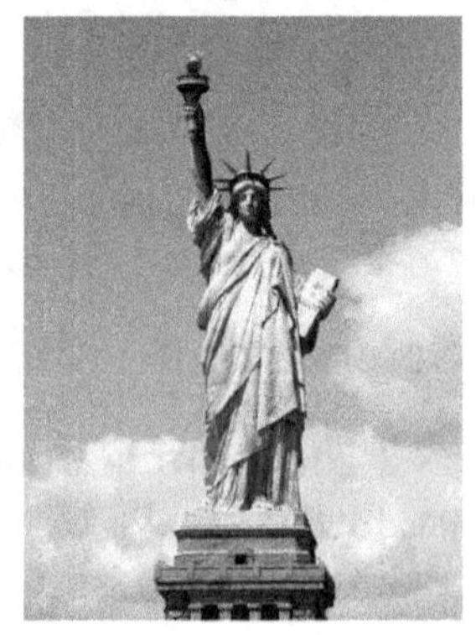 Cancer" in fraction of second. Beta-glucosidase enzyme only present in cancer cells, which triggers the unique cancer-destroying mechanism found in Vitamin B-17. Dr Burk also stated that evidence for Laetrile's efficacy had been noted in at least five independent institutions in three different countries.

Dr. Harold W. Manner, Professor of Biology and Chairman of the Biology Department of Chicago's Loyola University said, "I was lecturing in Buffalo, New York and after I had praised Laetrile's efficacy and its role in cancer treatment, a man stood up and said Dr. Manner, how can you make such statements. Did you forget that a little girl in upstate New York took her father's Laetrile tablets and died of cyanide poisoning. Just then a little lady stood up and told angrily, "Dr. Manner let me answer this gentleman. I think I am only entitled to because I am that little girl's mother. My daughter never touched her father's Laetrile tablets. The doctor, knowing the father was on Laetrile, marked down possible cyanide poisoning. At the hospital, doctor injected her Sodium Nitrite injection (the antidote of Cyanide), that killed my child. And yet that statement will continue to appear that she died of laetrile poisoning, even though they know it is a lie.

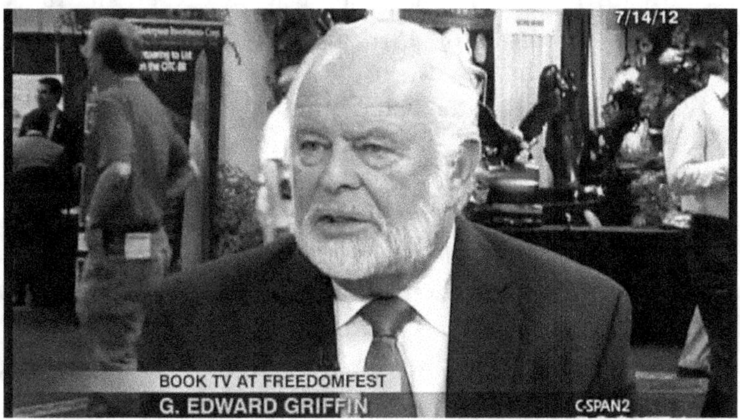

Dr. Ernesto Contreras operated the Oasis of Hope Hospital in Tijuana, Mexico for over 30 years. He has treated many thousands of cancer patients, most of them are American citizens. (World Without Cancer)

A drop from the ocean

(from the book "World Without Cancer" by G. Edward Griffin)

A great deal of drama has been enacted on the cancer stage since the first edition of this book was published. While it is true that many of the original actors have been replaced by their understudies, the plot of the play has not changed. This is the outline of that drama. Each year, thousands of Americans travel to Mexico and Germany to receive Laetrile therapy. They do this because it has been suppressed in the United States. Most of these patients have been told that their cancer is terminal and they have but a few months to live. Yet, an incredible percentage of them have recovered and are living normal lives. However, the FDA, the AMA, the American Cancer Society, and the cancer research centers continue to pronounce that Laetrile is quackery. The recovered patients, they say, either had "spontaneous remissions" or never had cancer in the first place. If any of these people ultimately die after seeking Laetrile, spokesmen for orthodox medicine are quick to proclaim: "You see? Laetrile doesn't work!" Meanwhile, hundreds of thousands of patients die each year after undergoing surgery, radiation, or chemotherapy, but those treatments continue to be touted as "safe and effective." The average cancer patient undergoing Laetrile therapy will spend between $5,000 and $25,000 for treatment. That is a lot of money, but it is peanuts compared to the astronomical bills charged by conventional medicine. Yet they never tire of complaining that Laetrile doctors are greedy quacks and charlatans who profiteer from the sick and the frightened. That is a classic case of accusing your opponent of exactly what you yourself are doing. It is common today for an elderly couple to give their entire life savings to a medical center and a battery of attending physicians and technicians, all in the vain hope of saving the husband or wife from cancer. Even their house may have to be sold to pay the bills. And the maddening part is that, in most cases, the doctors *know* there is no chance of long-term success. But the surviving spouse is seldom told that.

It has been suggested that the mass media have decided to ignore Laetrile because, when it did receive national publicity, it became popular. People decided to give it a try in spite of the negative press. If they had been told they were going to die anyway, why not? And the clinics in Mexico thrived. Each unfolding event is merely an extension of forces and arguments that have preceded. For example, in 1977, the parents of Chad Green kidnapped their own son and took him to Mexico to avoid being forced by officials in Massachusetts into giving him chemotherapy for his leukemia. They preferred nutritional therapy instead. This is part of the heavy price we pay for allowing government the power to decide what is best for us and our families. When special-interest groups become politically strong enough to write the laws, then it is *those groups* that tell us what to do-all in the name of protecting us, of course.

The Chad Green story made big headlines but, unfortunately, the same thing involving other children has happened numerous times since then with only minor news coverage. For example, in 1999, James and Donna Navarro were told that their four-year-old son, Thomas, had a malignant brain tumor. Surgery left the child speechless, blind, and unable to walk. When the doctors told the Navarros that Thomas would also have to undergo radiation and chemotherapy, they researched the medical literature and learned that these treatments probably would further impair the boys brain function and that long-term survival was unlikely anyway. So they decided to try an alternative therapy called *antineoplastons* offered at the Stanislaw R. Burzynsky Research Institute in Houston. At this point, the FDA stepped in and prohibited Dr. Burzynsky from accepting the boy as a patient unless he first had undergone chemotherapy and radiation. Mr. Navarro explains: "What they don't understand is that there won't be anything left of him to salvage if we make him take that awful treatment first." When he did not fall in line with the doctors' demands, he began to receive harassing phone calls from hospital personnel. One oncologist threatened to file charges with the state. When Mr. Navarro still refused, the doctor went to the protective-services agency and filed child abuse charges against the parents. - G. Edward Griffin (World Without Cancer)

World Without Cancer – Edward Griffin

This year 350,000 Americans will die from cancer. One out of four of us will develop cancer in our lifetime. That's over 50 million people in the United States alone.

The purpose of this presentation is to show that this great human tragedy can be stopped now entirely on the basis of existing scientific knowledge.

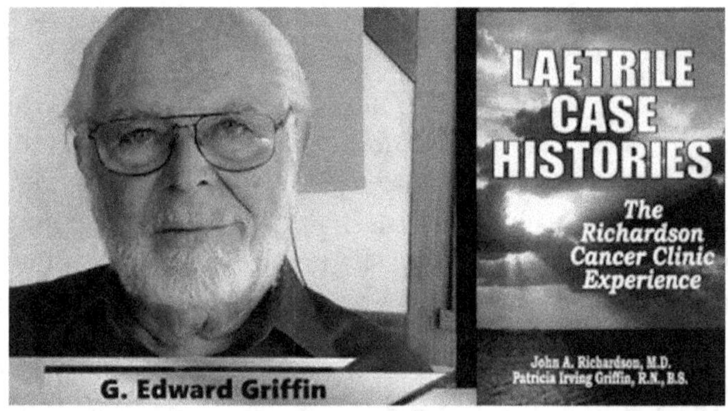

We'll explore the theory that cancer, like scurvy or pellagra, is a deficiency disease aggravated by the lack of an essential food compound in modern man's diet and that its ultimate control is to be found simply in restoring this substance to our daily intake.

We are not in the business of promoting vitamins, food supplements or products of any kind. We're not prescribing any course of treatment. We endorse nothing, except freedom of choice. We have nothing to sell, but facts.

What you're about to hear, does not carry the approval of organized medicine. The Food and Drug Administration, the American Cancer Society and the American Medical Association have labeled it fraud and quackery.

The average physician, however, is less dogmatic. He's more apt to say: "Let's give it a try and then pass judgement!" Consequently, an increasing number of doctors all over the world now are testing and proving in their own clinics that the vitamin concept of cancer is true.

With billions of dollars spent each year on research, with other billions taken in from the cancer-related sale of drugs and with vote-hungry politicians promising ever-increasing government programs we find that today there are more people making a living from cancer, than are dying from it. If the riddle were to be solved by a simple vitamin, this gigantic commercial and political industry could be wiped out overnight. The result is that the science of cancer therapy isn't nearly as complicated as the politics of cancer therapy.

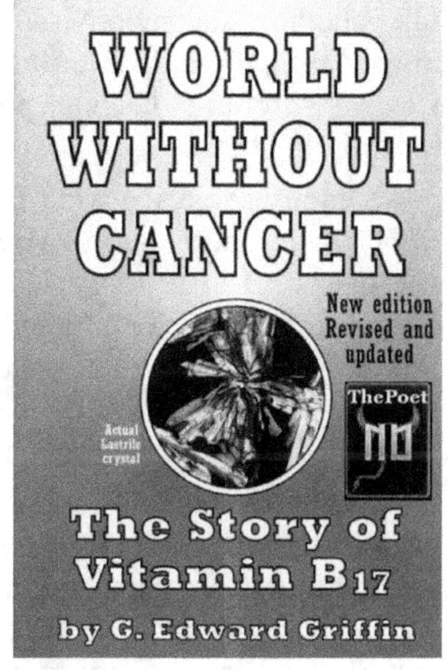

In the past the FDA and other agencies of government have used every means at their disposal to prevent this story from being told. They've arrested citizens for holding public meetings to tell others of their convictions on this subject. They've confiscated films and books. They even now are prosecuting doctors, who apply these theories in an effort to save the lives of their own patients.

With this background in mind it may appear to be the height of folly to proceed with this presentation. But ladies and gentlemen, if the story that follows is true, - as we firmly are convinced, it is - then in the name of humanity someone simply has to stand up against the bureaucracy and we are determined to do it!

The history of science is the history of struggle against entrenched error. Many of the world's greatest discoveries initially were rejected by the scientific community and those, who pioneered those discoveries, often were ridiculed and condemned as quacks and charlatans.

Columbus was bitterly attacked for believing, the Earth was round. Bruno was burned at the stake for claiming, the Earth was not the center of the universe. Galileo was imprisoned for teaching that the Earth moved around the Sun. Even the Wright brothers were ridiculed and condemned for claiming that a machine could fly above the Earth.

In the field of medicine Andreas Vesalius was denounced as an impostor and heretic because of his discoveries in the field of human anatomy. William Harvey was disgraced as a physician for believing that blood was pumped by the heart and actually moved around the body through arteries. And Ignaz Semmelweis was fired from his hospital post for requiring his maternity staff to wash their hands.

Centuries ago it wasn't unusual for entire naval expeditions to be wiped out by scurvy. Between 1600 and 1800 the casualty list of the British Navy alone was over one million sailors. Medical experts of the time were baffled, as they searched in vain for some kind of a strange bacterium, virus or toxin that supposedly lurked in the dark holds of ships. And yet for hundreds of years the cure was already known and written in the record.

In the winter of 1535, when the French explorer Jacques Cartier found his ships frozen in the ice off the St. Lawrence River, scurvy began to take its deadly toll. Out of a crew of one hundred and ten, twenty-five already had died and most of the others were so ill, they weren't expected to recover.

And then a friendly Indian showed them the simple remedy. Tree bark and needles from the white pine - both rich in ascorbic acid or vitamin C - were stirred into a drink, which produced immediate improvement and swift recovery.

Upon returning to Europe, Cartier reported this incident to the medical authorities. But they were amused by such "witch-doctor cures of ignorant savages" and they did nothing to follow it up.

Yes, the cure for scurvy was known. But because of scientific arrogance it took over two hundred years and cost hundreds of thousands of lives, before the medical experts began to accept and apply this knowledge.

Finally in 1747 John Lind, a young surgeon's mate in the British Navy discovered that oranges and lemons produced relief from scurvy and recommended that the Royal Navy include citrus fruits in the stores of all its ships. And yet, it still took forty-eight more years, before his recommendation was put into effect.

The twentieth century has proven to be no exception to this pattern. Only a generation ago large portions of the American Southeast were decimated by the dread disease of pellagra, which was thought to be contagious and probably caused by an as yet undiscovered virus. As far back as 1914 Dr. Joseph Goldberger had proven that this condition was related to diet and later showed that it could be prevented simply by eating liver or yeast. But it wasn't until the 1940s - almost thirty years later - that the medical world fully accepted pellagra as a vitamin B deficiency.

By 1952 Dr. Ernst T. Krebs, Jr., a biochemist in San Francisco, had advanced the theory that cancer, like scurvy or pellagra, is not caused by some kind of mysterious bacterium, virus or toxin, but is merely a deficiency disease aggravated by the lack of an essential food compound in modern man's diet. He identified this compound as part of the nitriloside family, which occurs abundantly in nature in over twelve hundred edible plants and found virtually in every part of the world. It's particularly prevalent in the seeds of fruits, but also is contained in grasses, maize, sorghum, millet, cassava, linseed, bitter almonds and many other foods that generally have been deleted from the menus of modern civilization.

A chronic disease is one, which usually doesn't pass away of its own accord. A metabolic disease is one, which arises within the body and isn't transmittable to another person. Cancer therefore is defined as a chronic, metabolic disease.

Dr. Krebs has pointed out that in the entire history of medical science there hasn't been one chronic, metabolic disease that was ever cured and prevented by drugs or mechanical manipulation of the body. In every case the ultimate solution was found only in factors relating to adequate nutrition. And he thinks that this is an important clue as to where to concentrate our scientific curiosity in the search for a better understanding of cancer.

But there are other clues, as well. Before looking at the more technical aspects of Dr. Krebs's theory, it's well that we examine some of them. For example, domesticated pets often seek out certain grasses to eat, even though they're adequately filled by other foods. This is particularly likely to happen, if the animals are not well. It's interesting to note that the grasses selected by instinct are Johnson grass, Tunis grass, Sudan grass and others that are especially rich in nitrilosides or vitamin B17.

Monkeys and other primates at the zoo, when given a fresh peach or apricot, will carefully pull away the sweet, fleshy part, crack open the hard pit and devour the small seed that remains. Instinct compels them to do this, even though they've never seen that kind of fruit before. These seeds are one of the most concentrated sources of nitrilosides to be found anywhere in nature.

Wild bears are great consumers of nitrilosides in their natural diet. Not only do they seek out berries that are rich in this substance, but when they kill small grazing animals for their own food, instinctively they pass over the muscle portions and consume first the viscera and rumen, which are filled with nitriloside grasses.

In captivity, animals seldom are allowed to eat all the foods of their instinctive choice. In the San Diego Zoo, for example, the routine diet for bears, although adequate in volume and nutritious in many other respects, is almost totally devoid of nitrilosides. In one grotto alone over a six-year period five bears died of cancer. It was generally speculated by the experts that a virus had been the cause.

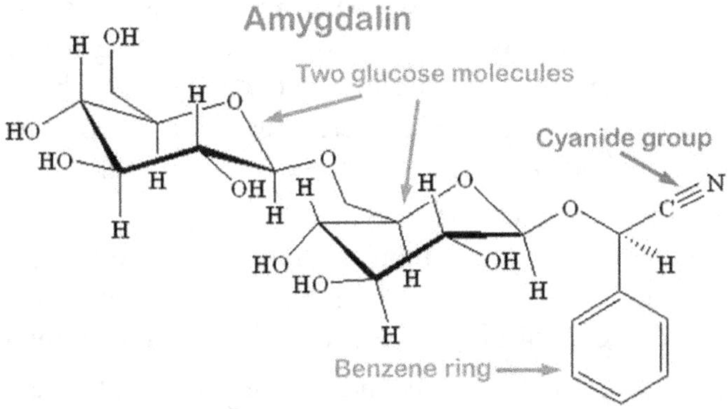

Now, it's highly significant that one never finds cancer in the carcasses of wild animals killed in the hunt. These creatures contract the disease only, when they are domesticated by man and forced to eat the foods that he provides and the scraps from his table.

Dr. George M. Briggs, professor of nutrition at the University of California has said: "The typical American diet is a national disaster... If I fed it to pigs or cows without adding vitamins and other supplements, I could wipe out the livestock industry."

A brief look at the American diet tells the story. Grocery shelves now are lined with high-carbohydrate foods that have been processed, refined, synthesized, artificially flavored and loaded with chemical preservatives. Some manufacturers even boast of how little real food there is in their product.

Millet once was the nation's staple grain. It is high in nitriloside content. But now it's been replaced by wheat, which has practically none at all. Sorghum cane has been replaced by sugar cane with the same result. Even our cattle are fed increasingly on quick-growing, low-nitriloside grasses, so there's less vitamin B17 residue in the meat we eat. In some places livestock now are being fed a diet containing fifteen percent paper to fatten them quicker for market.

And so we see that in the past 50 years the foods, that once provided the American people with ample amounts of natural vitamin B17, gradually have been pushed aside or replaced altogether by foods almost devoid of this factor. Significantly it's during this same time span that the cancer rate has moved steadily upward to the point, where today one out of every four persons in the United States is destined to contract this disease.

The ultimate scientific test of the vitamin theory of cancer would be to take a large number of people numbering in the thousands and over a period of many years expose them to a consistent diet of rich-nitriloside foods and then check the results.

Fortunately this already has been done. In the remote recesses of the Himalaya Mountains between West Pakistan, India and China there is a tiny kingdom called Hunza. These people are known world over for their amazing longevity and good health. It's not uncommon for Hunzakuts to live beyond a hundred years and some even to a hundred and twenty or more. Visiting medical teams from the outside world report that there never has been a case of cancer in Hunza.

Although presently accepted science is unable to explain, why these people should be free of cancer, it's interesting to note that the average Hunza diet contains over two-hundred times more nitriloside, than the average American diet. In fact, in that land, where there is no such thing as money, a man's wealth is measured by the number of apricot trees he owns. And the most prized of all foods is considered to be the apricot seed.

It's also interesting to learn that when the Hunzakuts leave their secluded land and adopt the menus of other countries, they soon succumb to the same diseases and infirmities - including cancer - as the rest of mankind.

The Eskimos are another people that have been observed by medical teams for many decades and found to be totally free of cancer. The traditional Eskimo diet is amazingly rich in nitrilosides that come from the residue in the meat of caribou and other grazing animals and also from the salmon berry, which grows abundantly in the Arctic areas.

When the Eskimo abandons his traditional way of life and begins to rely on westernized foods, he becomes even more cancer-prone, than the average American.

There are many other peoples in the world that could be cited with the same characteristics: the Abkhazians near the Black Sea, the Hopi and Navajo Indians of North America, certain native populations in South America and South Africa.

From all races and all regions of the world the one thing they have in common is that the degree, to which these people are free from cancer, is in direct proportion to the amount of nitrilosides or vitamin B17 found in their native diet.

In answer to this the skeptic may argue that these primitive groups aren't exposed to the same cancer-producing elements that modern man is and perhaps that's why they're immune. Let them breathe the same smog-filled air, smoke the same cigarettes, swallow the same chemicals added to their food or drinking water, use the same soaps or deodorants and then see, how they fare!

This, of course, is a valid point. But fortunately even that question now has been resolved by experience.

For over two decades there has been a steadily growing group of people, who have accepted the vitamin theory of cancer and who have altered their diets accordingly. They represent all walks of life, all ages, both sexes and reside in almost every advanced nation in the world. It's estimated that there are many thousands in the United States alone.

Now it's true that there's no way to determine their exact number or to conduct clinical examinations on each of them. But they do constitute a rather well defined group that is both vocal and conspicuous. It's significant therefore that after starting and maintaining a diet rich in vitamin B17 none of these people has ever been known to contract cancer.

Now let's repeat that statement! While their fellow citizens are suffering from cancer at the rate of one out of every four, not one of these thousands has ever been known to contract this dread disease.

For many persons the logic of all these facts put together is so great that it would be easy to close the case right here. But in view of the powerful opposition against this concept let's not content ourselves only with the logic of the theory! Let's reinforce our convictions with the science of the theory also, that we may understand, why it works the way, our logic tells us that it must.

In 1902 John Beard, a professor of embryology at the University of Edinburgh in Scotland, reported that there were no discernible differences between highly malignant cancer cells and certain pre-embryonic cells that were quite normal in the early stages of pregnancy. In technical terms these normal cells are called trophoblasts. Extensive research had led Professor Beard to the conclusion that cancer and trophoblast are in fact one and the same. His theory therefore is known as the trophoblastic thesis of cancer.

The trophoblast in pregnancy indeed does exhibit all the classical characteristics of cancer. It spreads and multiplies rapidly, as it eats its way into the uterus wall preparing a place, where the embryo can attach itself for maternal protection and nourishment.

The trophoblast is formed as a result of a chain reaction starting with another cell identified as the diploid totipotent. For our purposes let's call this simply the "total-life" cell, because it contains within it all the separate characteristics of the complete organism and has the total capacity to evolve into any organ or tissue or for that matter into the complete embryo itself.

About eighty percent of these total-life cells are located in the ovaries or testes, where they serve as a genetic reservoir for future offspring. The rest of them are distributed elsewhere in the body for a purpose not yet fully understood, but which may involve the regenerative or healing process of damaged tissue.

The hormone estrogen is well known for its ability to effect changes in living tissue. Although it's generally thought of as a female hormone, it's found in both sexes and performs many vital functions. Wherever the body is damaged either by physical trauma, chemical action or illness, estrogen always appears in great quantities, possibly serving as a stimulator or catalyst for body repair.

It's now known that the total-life cell is triggered into producing trophoblast, when it comes into contact with estrogen. When this happens to those total-life cells that have evolved from the ferilized egg, the result is a placenta and umbilical cord, a means of nourishing the embryo. But when it occurs non-sexually as part of the general healing process, the result is cancer.

When cancer begins to form, the body reacts by attempting to seal it off and surrounding it with cells that are similar to those in the location, where it occurs. A bump or lump is the usual result.

Under microscopic examination most of these tumors are found to resemble a mixture or hybrid of both trophoblast and surrounding cells; a fact, which has led many researchers to the premature conclusion that there are many different types of cancer. But the degree, to which various tumors appear to be different, is the same degree, to which they're benign; which means that it's the degree, to which there are non-cancerous cells within it.

The greater the malignancy, the more these tumors begin to resemble each other and the more clearly they begin to take on the classic characteristics of pregnancy trophoblast. And the most malignant of all cancers, the chorionepitheliomas, are almost indistinguishable from trophoblast cells. For, as Dr. Beard pointed out over seventy years ago, they're one and the same.

Let's turn now to the question of defense mechanisms! Before we can hope to conquer cancer, first we must understand, how nature conquers cancer, how nature protects, the body and controls the growth of trophoblast cells.

All animals contain billions of white blood cells. One of the functions of these cells is to attack and destroy anything that is foreign and harmful to our bodies.

For this reason it would seem logical that they would attack cancer cells, also.

But since cancer is trophoblast and since trophoblast is not foreign to the body, but is in fact a vital part of the life cycle, nature has provided it with a very effective means of avoiding the white cells.

One of the characteristics of the trophoblast is that it's surrounded by a thin protein coating that carries a negative electrostatic charge. The white cells also have a negative charge. And since similar polarities repel each other, the trophoblast is well protected.

Part of the solution to this problem is found in the pancreas, which secretes an enzyme called trypsin. When this enzyme reaches the trophoblast in sufficient quantity, it digests the protective protein coat. The cancer then is exposed to the attack of the white cells and it dies.

Applying this to the embryo we find that the trophoblast cells there continue to grow and spread right up to the eighth week. And then suddenly with no apparent reason they stop growing and are destroyed. Recent research has provided the explanation. It's in the eighth week that the baby's pancreas begins to function.

Now it's significant that the upper intestines - near the point, where the pancreas empties into it - is the one place in the human body, where cancer is almost never found.

We note also that diabetics - those, who suffer from a pancreas malfunction - are three times more likely to contract cancer, than non-diabetics.

These facts, which have puzzled medical investigators for years, at last can be explained in light of the trophoblastic thesis of cancer.

But what happens, if the pancreas is weak or if the rate of cancer growth is so high that the enzyme trypsin can't keep up with it? Then what?

The answer is that nature has provided a backup mechanism, a second line of defense, that can do the job, even if the first line should fail. It involves a unique chemical compound that poisons the malignant cell, while nourishing all the rest. And this is, where the vitamin concept of cancer finally comes back into the picture.

The chemical compound in question, of course, is vitamin B17, which is found in those natural foods containing nitrilosides. It's known also as amygdalin and as such has been used and studied extensively for well over a hundred years. But in its concentrated and purified form developed by Dr. Krebs specifically for cancer therapy it is known as Laetrile. For the sake of clarity in this presentation, however, we shall favor the more simple name: vitamin B17.

The B17 molecule contains two units of sugar, one of benzaldehyde and one of cyanide, all tightly locked together within it. Now, as everyone knows, cyanide can be highly toxic and even fatal, if taken in sufficient quantity. However, locked as it is in this natural state, it's completely inert chemically and has absolutely no effect on living tissue.

There is only one substance that can unlock this molecule and release the cyanide. That substance is an enzyme called beta-glucosidase, which we shall call the "unlocking enzyme". When B17 comes in contact with this enzyme, not only is the cyanide released, but also the benzaldehyde, which is highly toxic by itself. In fact, these two working together are at least one hundred times more poisonous, than either of them separately.

The unlocking enzyme is not found to any dangerous degree anywhere in the body, except at the cancer cell, where it always is present in great quantity. The result is that vitamin B17 is unlocked at the cancer cell. It becomes poisonous to the cancer cell and only to the cancer cell.

There's another important enzyme called rhodanese, which we shall identify as the "protecting enzyme. The reason is that it has the ability to neutralize cyanide by converting it instantly into by-products that actually are beneficial and essential for health. This enzyme is found in great quantities in every part of the body, except the cancer cell, which consequently is not protected.

Here then is a biochemical process that destroys cancer cells, while at the same time nourishes and sustains non-cancer cells. It's an intricate and perfect mechanism of nature that simply couldn't have been accidental.

There's much speculation today about carcinogens, the things that supposedly cause cancer. We're told that researchers now have proven that smoking or excessive exposure to the sun or chemical additives to our food or even certain viruses all can cause cancer. But as we have seen, the real cause is an enzyme and vitamin deficiency. These other things merely are the specific triggers that start the process.

Anything that producess prolonged stress or damage to the body can trigger off the production of estrogen as a part of the healing process. If this goes unchecked, because the body lacks the necessary chemical ingredients to fight back, then the result is cancer.

Specific carcinogens therefore do not cause cancer. They merely determine, where it's going to occur.

Of course, nature's defenses against cancer include more, than just the pancreatic enzymes and vitamin B17.

Research has shown that an important role also may be played by other enzymes, other vitamins, oxygenation of the blood, pH levels and even body temperature. Vitamin B17 seems to be the most vital and direct-acting of all these factors, but none of them can be ignored, for they're an interlocking part of the total natural mechanism.

Fortunately, it's not necessary for man to understand fully every theoretical aspect of this mechanism, in order to make it work for him in practice. All that he really needs to know is the necessity of eating foods rich in all the vitamins and minerals and of minimizing damage or stress to the body.

The reality of the vitamin B17 concept of cancer has been proven in the laboratory beyond any doubt. For example, Dr. Dean Burk, head of the Cytochemistry Section of the National Cancer Institute, has reported that in a series of tests on animal tissue the B17 had no effect on normal cells, but released so much cyanide and benzaldehyde, when it came in contact with cancer cells that not one of them could survive. He said: "When we add Laetrile to a cancer culture under the microscope, we can see the cancer cells dying off like flies."

We've said that vitamin B17 is harmless to non-cancer cells. This is true, but perhaps it would be more accurate to say that it's as harmless as any substance can be. After all, even life-essential water or oxygen can be fatal, if taken in unnaturally large doses. And this is true also of vitamin B17.

For example, there's one case of a man, who reportedly died from devouring almost a cup of apple seeds. Incidentally, the case never has been authenticated, but assuming it's true, if the man had eaten the apples also, he would have obtained enough extra rhodanese from the whole fruit to offset the effect of even that many seeds in his stomach. But that would have required that he eat several cases of apples, which, of course, would have been impossible in the first place.

Nature can only do so much. It cannot anticipate excess of this kind. Therefore it's wise to follow the simple rule that one should not eat at one time more seeds, than he likely would consume, if he also were eating a reasonable quantity of the whole fruit. This is a common-sense rule with a large safety margin that can be followed with complete confidence.

Therapies and Protocols (Metabolic Therapy)

Phase 1 - The First 21 Days

The initial phase consists of a 21-day therapy in which clinics include the intravenous form of B17, sometimes combined with the tissue-penetrating agent DMSO and high doses of Vitamin C. However 500mg amygdalin (B17) tablets, together with apricot kernels, are often employed for home use if intravenous treatment is not available. Supplementary therapies in Phase 1 include pancreatic enzymes, Vitamin C, antioxidants, emulsified vitamins A & E, Barley Green powder, shark cartilage (100% pure), multivitamins, Pangamic Acid (vitamin B-15), AHCC and actual whole foods that contain B17 (e.g. apricot seeds). Detoxification and full nutritional supplementation procedures are also rigorously followed.

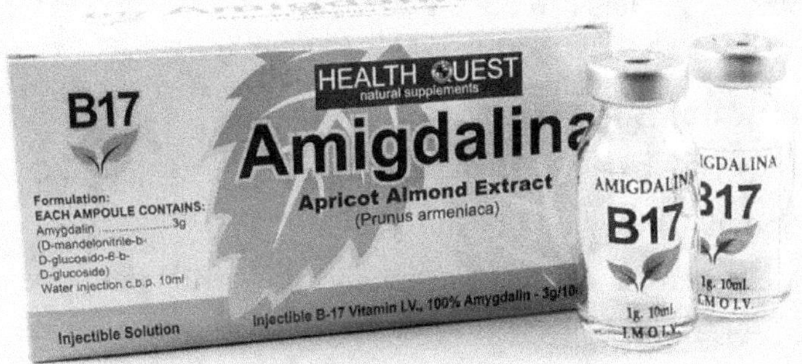

Phase 2 - The Next 3 Months

The second phase consists of Vitamin B 17/amygdalin tablets, apricot seeds, enzymes, Vitamins A, C and E, shark cartilage and the continuing detoxification and nutritional procedures initiated in Phase 1.

Phase I Metabolic for the first 21 days

Phase I Intravenous

(Obtained from The Physician's Handbook of Vitamin B17 Therapy)

Amygdalin injections: Two vials of Laetrile is given IV three times weekly for three weeks with at least one day between injections (Mon., Wed., Fri.). Dose of Amygdalin Tablets 500 mg is 2 tab three times a day with meals on the days on which the patients do not receive the intravenous Laetrile. Warm the injection vials by putting them in a bowl of lukewarm water for 2-3 minutes.

The dosage for the intravenous Laetrile is:

1st dose 1 vial (10 cc- 3 gms.)
2nd dose 2 vials (20 cc- 6 gms.)
3rd dose 2 vials (20 cc- 6 gms.)
4th through the 9th dose 3 vials (30 cc-9 gms.)

Nutritional Supplements:

- Vitamin B15 (pangamic acid): One capsule three times a daily at the end of each meal.

- Preven-ca capsules (contains powerful antioxidants and herbs): One capsule with each meal.

- Megazyme Forte enzyme tablets: Three tablets two hours after each meal (9 daily).

- Ester C (Vitamin C) tablets: One capsule with each meal.

- Vitamin A & E emulsion drops: 5 drops in juice or water three times per day.

- Just Barley Green Juice (nutritional supplement): One teaspoon in juice three times per day.

- Shark cartilage: 3 capsules with each meal (9 daily).

- Vitamin E: One gel with lunch and one with dinner.

- AHCC (Active Hexose Correlated Compound): Two capsules with each meal.

- Daily Complete liquid multivitamin Nutrient: 1 oz (two tablespoons) once daily with a meal.

- Apricot kernels: One apricot kernel for every 10 lbs of body weight. No more than 6 per hour or 30-35 per day is recommended.

Not included is DMSO (dimethyl sulfoxide) for IV administration (some doctors use this compound to achieve fuller penetration of the B17).

OR

Phase I Oral

Injectable/IV Amygdalin is replaced with 500mg Amygdalin tablets. Dr. Contreras recommends 2 of these tablets with each meal for a total of 6 per day. Otherwise the ORAL Phase 1 includes the same materials as above.

- **Vitamin B17 500 mg tablets:** 2 tablets three times daily with meals (6 daily). This is the most convenient and most frequently used method of Amygdalin administration. The tablet size is 500mg. If you have difficulty swallowing, the tablets may be broken up and added to soft food. If there is a gastric disturbance, then you should take one tablet six times daily. If you find that you are getting nauseous cut the tablets in half and have one every waking hour. It is a good idea to have some food in the stomach just before taking the vitamin.

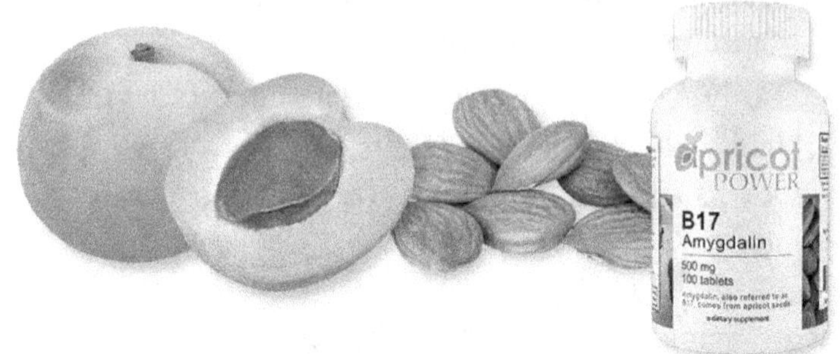

- Vitamin B15 (pangamic acid): One capsule three times a daily at the end of each meal.

- Preven-ca capsules (contains powerful antioxidants and herbs): One capsule with each meal.

- Megazyme Forte enzyme tablets: Three tablets two hours after each meal (9 daily).

- Ester C (Vitamin C) tablets: One capsule with each meal.

- Vitamin A & E emulsion drops: 5 drops in juice or water three times per day.

- Barley Green Juice (nutritional supplement): One teaspoon in juice three times per day.

- Shark cartilage: 3 capsules with each meal (9 daily).

- Vitamin E: One gel with lunch and one with dinner.

- AHCC (Active Hexose Correlated Compound): Two capsules with each meal.

- Daily Complete liquid multivitamin Nutrient: 1 oz (two tablespoons) once daily with a meal.

- Apricot kernels: One apricot kernel for every 10 lbs of body weight. No more than 6 per hour or 30-35 per day is recommended.

Then, after the first 21 days….

Phase 2 for the next 3 months

Pack comprises B17 in 500mg tablet form with the same materials as Phase 1 except that the dosages for the vitamin B17 as well as the A&E Emulsion Drops change to the following:

- Vitamin B17 500 mg tablets: 1 tablet with each meal and one at bedtime.

- Vitamin A & E emulsion drops: 10 drops in juice or water two times per day (suspend for 2 months after 3 months of use).

Costs range from £490.00 to £650.00 for Phase I (1st 21 days) and £1,320.00 to £1,500.00 for Phase II (subsequent 3 months)

Most distributors make these products available individually. Please be advised that distributors of metabolic therapy products may not answer individual medical questions nor give specific information about the therapeutic use of any of their products. These products are regarded only as food supplements for daily nutritional supplementation.

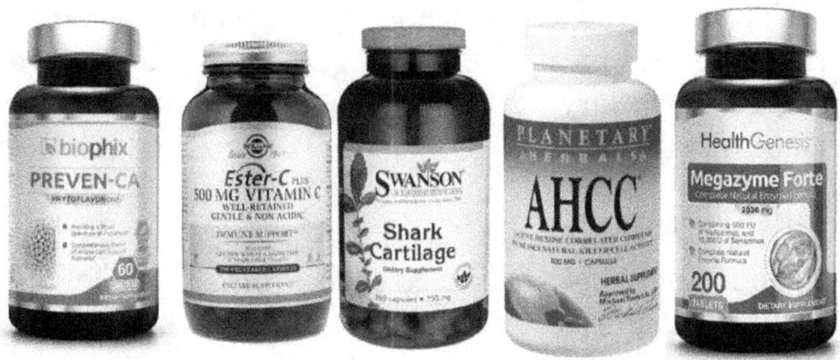

Maintenance Dosage

Obtained from The Physician's Handbook of Vitamin B17 Therapy

Dr. Krebs suggests that over a period of time a total dosage in excess of 300 grams is the average in controlling a moderate cancer crisis. The time needed to develop the maximum response is four months to over a year. If good response is obtained within the first three weeks, the dosage may be reduced or the clinical schedule changed to suit the convenience of the patient.

A severe cancer crisis brought under control may be maintained in a quiescent state by the oral administration of 1 gram of Vitamin B-17 daily. However some patients claim to feel "better" or "safer" with 1.5 to 2.0 grams daily. Such dosage is determined by the patient's sense of well being, gain in strength, increased appetite, weight gain, and psychological improvement with reduction of anxiety and nervousness, with exhibition of a more nearly normal degree of optimism and interest in his environment.

Abnormal situations, stress or ill health of any kind have been known to be followed by a renewed outbreak or progression of the cancer process in some patients. The attending physician should be aware of these possibilities with patients in whom the cancer is under control. When a cancer crisis has been successfully controlled for more than two years, with patient showing good objective responses in weight gain, increased strength, return to a more nearly normal state of activity and vigor, with negative CGH urine tests, and with an improvement in x-rays or other objective evidence, the maintenance dose may be reduced to dietary levels of vitamin B17 of at least 500 milligrams per day.

Precautions

- Following this first three weeks of I.V. injections, the patient then has one injection of 1 vial (10cc-3 gms.) once weekly for three months. But if the patient notices a considerable difference in the way he feels when the injections are reduced to once weekly, the injections are again increased to two or three times a week for three weeks. The dose is then reduced again to once weekly. This is repeated as often as necessary until the patient notices no difference with the reduced dosage.

- The oral Laetrile is given in a dosage of 1 gram (two 500 mg. tablets) daily on the days on which the patients do not receive the intravenous Laetrile. Ask the patient to take both tablets at the same time at bedtime on an empty stomach with water. The water is important because there are some enzymes in the fruits and vegetables and in their juices which will destroy part of the potency of the Laetrile tablets while they are in the stomach. Once the stomach has emptied, this is no problem.

- It should be noted that do not start the Laetrile, either I.V. or orally, until the patients have been on their vitamins, enzymes and diet for a period of ten days to two weeks. Laetrile seems to have little or no effect until a sufficient quantity of other vitamins and minerals are in the body. Zinc, for example, is the transportation mechanism for the Laetrile. In the absence of sufficient quantities of zinc, the Laetrile does not get into the tissues. The body will not rebuild any tissue without sufficient quantities of Vitamin C, etc.

- When you start the intravenous and oral dosages of Laetrile, you also begin to increase the amount of Vitamin C. Increase their Vitamin C by one gram every third day until they reach a level of at least six grams. In some patients you need more. There are some patients who develop irritation of the stomach or diarrhea with the larger doses of Vitamin C. If these symptoms develop, reduce the Vitamin C to a level that causes no problem. Remember that most of the patients tolerate the higher doses of Vitamin C very well.

- On the days that my patients receive intravenous Laetrile, do not take Vitamin A & E. There have been some studies indicating that Vitamin A may interfere with the body's ability to metabolize intravenous Laetrile, though this has not been fully proved.

- Also, do not to take the Laetrile tablets on the days that you receive intravenous Laetrile. They have received intravenously as much Laetrile as the body can handle for that period of time. There are no ill effects from taking the tablets on those days, but the effect of the tablets is wasted.

- The level of nitrilosides in the body can be monitored. When the body metabolizes nitrilosides, the by-product is thiocyanate. Thiocyanate levels in the blood can be measured. Most of the patients who do best are those in whom the thiocyanate level is between 1.2 and 2.5 Mg/dl. This level can be raised or lowered by increasing or decreasing the dosage of the Laetrile tablets.

- Keep in mind that Laetrile is not the only source of nitrilosides. There are some 1500 foods that contain nitrilosides. These include apricot kernels, peach kernels, grape seeds, blackberries, blueberries, strawberries, bean sprouts, lima beans, and macadamia nuts. The advantage of using Laetrile in the cancer patient is that Laetrile is a concentrated form of nitrilosides. It can raise the nitriloside level in the body (and, thus, re-establish the body's second line of defense against cancer) much more rapidly than can be done by diet alone.

Metabolic Therapy Component Descriptions

- Injectable B17
- B17 (Amygdalin) Tablets
- Megazyme Forte
- Emulsified Vitamin A+E
- Shark Cartilage
- Apricot Kernels (Seeds)
- Vitamin B-15 (Pangamic Acid)
- Vitamin C (Esterfied)
- Active Hexose Correlated Compound (AHCC®)
- Vitamin E (d-alpha tocopherol acetate)

- PrevenCA Antioxidant Formula®
- Daily Complete Multi Vitamin
- Barley Grass (Just Barley® Juice)

Accessory Metabolic Supplements (Not routinely prescribed but recommended)

- Maximol (Neways International)
- Revenol (Neways International)
- Cascading Revenol
- Cassie-Tea (Neways International)
- Hawaiian Noni Juice (Neways International)
- Purge / Feelin' Good (Neways International)
- Dimethyl sulfoxide (DMSO)

Injectable (IV) B-17/Laetrile/Amygdalin

In Mexico, vitamin B-17 in metabolic therapy is administered through intravenous injection for the initial 21 days (phase I) of treatment and then orally afterwards (Phase II). 6 to 9 grams per day are used for the first 21 days in the Oasis of Hope hospital. Dr. Harold Manner and Dr. Ernsto Contreras used this protocol. Injectable B-17 is also invariably administered along with the tissue penetrating agent dimethyl Sulfoxide (DMSO).

Please Note: Clinical tests have repeatedly shown that vitamin B-17 is only truly effective when used in conjunction with pancreatic enzymes to break down the pericellular coating of the malignant cell. Vitamins A and E in their emulsified form, along with high doses of vitamin C, vitamin B-15, antioxidants, and other nutrients are then used in combination with B-17 to attack the cancer cell. Clinics administering Metabolic Therapy to their patients always use these supplements.

B-17/Laetrile/Amygdalin Tablets

Oral administration of Vitamin B-17 is the most convenient and frequently used method. These tablets contain the active B-17 ingredient derived from the kernels of apricots. Usually available in 100 mg or 500 mg tablets. These tablets are always taken in conjunction with the apricot seeds. Dr. Contreras recommends 2-4 100 mg tablets as a nutritional supplement for prevention. **4-6 500 mg tablets per day** as a nutritional supplement for clinical cancer sufferers, taken in conjunction with enzymes, antioxidants, and other supplements.

Dr. Krebs says "For some patients in whom gastric acidity is deficient, side reactions of weakness or headache following oral administration may be avoided by taking citrus juices or grape juice, or hydrochloric acid tablets such as betaine hydrochloride to prevent these unpleasant reactions".

Megazyme Forte Enzyme Supplement

Pancreatic enzyme preparations containing trypsin and chymotrypsin are included as an essential part of vitamin B-17 therapy. Oral dosage of pancreatic enzyme preparations is usually three tablets three times daily two hours after each meal for a total of nine tablets each day. Bromelain is also included in the therapeutic regimen for its proteolytic effect, and for a possible synergistic effect suggested by Dr. Nieper as occurring with vitamin B-17. Dr. Ernst T. Krebs also states: "The demasking effect of these enzymes against the pericellular layer of the malignant cell is something very concrete in the immunology of cancer. Now I prefer, rather than advising the use of bromelain or papaya tablets, that the individual seeking these enzymes get them directly from the fresh ripe pineapple and papaya fruit. As much as half a pineapple a day should be ingested".

The enzyme preparations recommended by Dr. Krebs, Dr. Hans Nieper, and Dr. Philip Binzel should be pH-sensitive and enteric coated. Ideally, they also should contain the following ingredients:

Pancreatin....…...................1250mg
Papain..........................150mg
Bromelain....................…....150mg
Trypsin..................…..........125mg
Lipase...................…...........50mg

Amylase...................................50mg
a-chymotrypsin.........................45mg
Rutin......................................100mg
Raw calf thymus concentrate....55mg
Zinc gluconate.........................10mg
Super oxide dismutase.............50mcg
Catalase..................................200 Units
L-Glutathione.........................10mg

Emulsified Vitamin A

In 1963 when Dr. Ernsto Contreras initiated his activities as a clinical oncologist, the use of Vitamin A as a useful agent in malignant neoplasm was considered illogical and absurd. Now, Vitamin-A is accepted as an agent of great use for the major epithelial cancers as well as for epidermis carcinomas, chronic leukemia and transitional cells.

The first formal studies of the possible anti-tumor effects of Vitamin A were initiated in Germany, by investigators of Mucos Laboratories in Munich. It was a proven fact, that lung cancer in Norwegian sailors was less common than in other groups, even though they smoked since childhood. Logic indicated that it had to be the opposite. After studying the Phenomenon, it was discovered that they ate abundant quantities of raw fish liver, high in Vitamin A, since childhood. The logical conclusion was that high doses of such vitamin prevented the growth of lung cancer in heavy smokers. But it was also found that high doses of Vitamin A were toxic, and could cause adverse reactions.

The main focus was to find out how to administer enough Vitamin A to observe preventive or healing effects, without injuring the liver. The solution was found by one of the investigators, when he discovered that unprocessed milk had the vitamin, and children who were breast-fed never experienced toxic effects. Nature had the solution by including Vitamin A in milk in the form of Micro-Emulsification.

Mucos investigators proceeded to prepare a variety of emulsified concentrations, formulating their famous High Concentration A-Mulsin. One drop contains 15,000 units. They were able to administer over a million units per day in progressive doses, without producing hepatic toxicity. The explanation is that, in emulsified form, Vitamin A is absorbed directly into the lymphatic system without going through the liver in high quantities. Having solved the toxicity problem, it was possible to test the product in high doses. It was demonstrated that Vitamin A has the following effects:

1. In normal doses, it protects epithelium and vision.

2. In doses of 100,000 to 300,000 units per day, it works as a potent immune stimulant.

3. In doses of 500,000 to 1,000,000 units per day, it works as a potent anti-tumor agent, especially in epidermis and transitional carcinomas.

Shark Cartilage

It has been said that sharks are the healthiest beings on earth. Sharks are immune to practically every disease known to man. Many scientists believe that the shark's skeleton, composed entirely of cartilage, is what is responsible for its incredible immunity to disease.

According to Dr. Contreras, when administered to cancer patients, shark cartilage has been reported to inhibit the growth of blood vessels, thereby restricting the vitality of the cancerous tumor. In addition, shark cartilage stimulates the production of antibodies and boosts the immune system. Not only is this a non-toxic product recommended for the treatment of cancer, but also for the treatment of inflammatory diseases such as rheumatism and osteoarthritis. Tumors are reported frequently to experience significant reduction in size within one to three months of the initial treatment. It is also noted to enhance the efficacy of vitamin B-17/amygdalin. For in depth information about shark cartilage, Jaws of Life by Dr. Alex Duarte and Sharks Don't Get Cancer by Dr. William Lane provide the complete story. Shark cartilage may be contra-indicated with pregnant or lactating women.

Apricot Seeds/Kernels

Apricot kernels are an inexpensive, rich and natural source of vitamin B-17. They also deliver the vitamins, minerals and enzymes not found in the pharmaceutical derivative of B-17.

- 10 seeds per day for life are recommended by Dr. Krebs as a nutritional supplement for those exercising cancer prevention.

- 30 to 35 seeds per day are recommended by Dr. Krebs as nutritional support for clinical cancer sufferers.

- In a minority of cases, cancer sufferers may experience nausea when taking seeds. In this event, clinics recommend that dosage is reduced and gradually increased as tolerance is gained. Not all apricot kernels are effective. They must have the characteristic bitter taste indicating that the B-17 ingredient is present. Not to be eaten whole. May be pulped, grated, or crushed.

Please note: Some cancer sufferers believe that apricot kernels alone are all that is required to fight cancer. Consultation with a qualified health practitioner familiar with Metabolic Therapy is advised for further information. Apricot kernels are usually part of the nutritional support for those exercising cancer prevention for life as well as cancer patients undergoing Phase 1 or Phase 2 Metabolic Therapy.

Vitamin B15 (Pangamic Acid)

Like B17, it too was discovered by Dr. E.T. Krebs, Jr. while exploring the chemical properties of apricot kernels in 1952. It could be said that it was an unexpected bonus or by-product of the search for vitamin B17. "The best way to understand the effect of vitamin B15 is to think of it as instant oxygen" says Dr. Krebs. "It increases the oxygen efficiency of the entire body and aids in the detoxification of waste products. Since cancer cells do not thrive in the presence of oxygen but depend rather on fermentation of glucose, it is probable that B15, indirectly, is an enemy of cancer".

In 1965 the U.S.S.R. Academy of Sciences released a 205-page symposium of its findings up to that date. In 1968 the Scientific Advisory Committee of the Ministry of Health unanimously ratified all the original claims in the report and authorized the Soviet drug industry to begin mass-production of B15 for general use. It has been reported that the Russian athletes have been given heavy doses of B15 during their participation at the Olympics. If this is true, there is good reason for it. Experiments have shown that this substance, although just a natural food factor, greatly increases physical strength and stamina. When rats were put into tubs of water and forced to swim, those that had received vitamin B15 were all still swimming long after the others had fatigued and drowned. When other rats were put into glass chambers from which oxygen gradually was removed, those that had received vitamins lived much longer-thus on less oxygen-than the control group.

The Soviet scientists disclosed that vitamin B15 is effective in such areas as circulatory problems, heart conditions, elevated blood cholesterol, skin disorders, hardening of the arteries, bronchial asthma, diabetes mellitus, and wound healing. They were especially emphatic in their findings that B15 was effective in retarding the ageing process! Professor Shpirt of the City Clinical Hospital No. 60 in Moscow concluded: "I believe the time will come when there will be calcium pangamate (B15) next to the salt shaker on the table of every family with people past forty."

Vitamin C (Esterfied)

Low levels of ascorbic acid intake may be associated with higher risks of cancer, heart disease and macular degeneration in the eyes of elderly persons. These are far more significant problems than the deadly disease this vitamin was first known to prevent, scurvy. Ester-C is a formula is designed to strengthen the immune system as well as work as an antioxidant and detoxifier. 99.9% of all animals in the world produce their own Vitamin C in the form of Mineral Ascorbates. Unfortunately, humans suffer from a genetic defect, hypoascorbemia, an inability to produce Vitamin C in our own bodies. Only a few other animals are known to share this problem with humans: Guinea pigs, monkeys, apes, and a type of bat. This may greatly explain why humans don't live so long as they might. A dog matures at 2 years and lives at least 7 times his period of maturity, or 14 years. Humans mature at 20 to 25 years. Seven times 20 equals 140 years, which would appear to be our life potential, if we could produce ascorbate in our own bodies.

In addition, reprints of articles published by metabolic physicians Dr. Ernst Krebs, Jr., Dr. Dean Burk (USA), Dr. Hans Nieper of Germany, Dr. Ernsto Contreras of Mexico, Dr. Manuel Navarro of the Philippines, and Dr. Shigeaki Sakai of Japan, concluded that nothing heals within the body without sufficient Vitamin C.

Ester-C is a Unique form of buffered vitamin C with metabolites. Metabolites are compounds derived from nutrients that are normally created in the body. Research has demonstrated that this combination of non-acidic C with metabolites is well absorbed and retained in blood cells and tissues. This product is further enhanced with the synergistic blend of bioflavonoids, acerola, rose hips, and rutin.

The unique, natural process produces a patented new form of Vitamin C which is gentle to the stomach, non-acidic, with a neutral pH. The only form of C containing natural metabolites to enhance bioavailability of Vitamin C.

Active Hexose Correlated Compound (AHCC)

AHCC (Active Hexose Correlated Compound) is an extract obtained from a hybridization of several kinds of mushrooms, which are grown in a liquid medium. AHCC contains naturally occurring beneficial ingredients called oligosaccharides (alpha -

1- 4 glucan), activated hemicellulose, amino acids, and glycoproteins.

Clinical tests have shown that AHCC can be a promising nutritional supplement to traditional anticancer Protocols. It has proven to help increase overall effectiveness while reducing many of the common side effects and improving overall quality of life. According to researchers at the Hokkaido, Kyorin, and Teikyo Universities in Japan, AHCC works by creating a stronger immune response throughout the body. They concluded that it increases the production of NK cells, Killer T-cells, and it induces the production of cytokine. They also concluded that AHCC helps induce levels of Interferon-Gamma, IL-12, IL-2, and TNF-Alpha and it inhibits lAP and TGF-beta. Research is still underway to discover the actual mechanism and how this precisely happens.

AHCC has also started to attract attention in North America. A study was recently conducted at the Oasis of Hope Hospital in Mexico, which produced favorable results. The University of California recently conducted a six-month study in which prostate cancer patients were given 9 grams of AHCC per day. The Southwest College of Naturopathic Medicine recently started a six-month trial involving HIV/AIDS patients. In addition to these two formal clinical trials, numerous other physicians and several major research institutes including Columbia University have been working with AHCC on an informal basis. Clinical trials using AHCC treatment for AIDS and HIV patients are also currently being conducted.

Vitamin E (d-alpha tocopherol acetate)

Vitamin E is a powerful antioxidant that protects cell membranes as well as other parts of the body, which are fat-soluble. Dr. Philip Binzel describes its therapeutic use with vitamin B17 in his book Alive and Well. Dr. Krebs, in his book The Physician's Handbook of Vitamin B-17 Therapy describes it as follows: "Vitamin E may augment the anti-oxidant effect of Vitamin C and aid in the conservation of oxygen in tissues.

Patients with elevated blood pressure should be started on small doses gradually increased as blood pressure adaptation occurs*. The dosage range is from 300 to 2400 I.U. per day."

Preven-CA Antioxidant Formula

Preven-CA is a natural source of important nutrients that contain powerful antioxidants and other substances with great protective and preventive value. Antioxidants neutralise cell damage caused by free radicals, formed by high fat diets, smoking, smog, alcohol, ultraviolet radiation, and other many other substances generated in our modern lifestyles. Many cancer patients have taken this product as aid in their treatments and it is now widely used in USA, Japan, and Mexico.

Preven-ca is a combination of shark cartilage and medicinal herbs, which contains many essential amino acids. It was designed by the OASIS doctors to inhibit tumor growth, provide antioxidants to detoxify the body, strengthen the immune system, and provide to important nutrients complement the patient's daily nutrition.

Preven-ca is a natural formula for prevention containing the following elements:

Cardus Marianus: Also known as milk thistle extract. It may protect the cells of the liver by blocking the entrance of harmful toxins and helping remove these toxins from the liver cells. As with other bioflavonoids, cardius marianus is a powerful antioxidant. It also regenerates injured liver cells. Milk thistle extract is most commonly recommended to counteract the harmful actions of alcohol on the liver. This substance has no side effects.

Grape Seed Extract: The main functions of proanthocyanidins (found in grape seed extract) are antioxidant activity, stabilization of collagen, and maintenance of elastin- two critical proteins in connective tissue, blood vessels, and muscle.

Carrot Root: It acts as an antioxidant and immune system booster.

Vitamins: A (20,000 I.U.), vitamins B-1, B-2, B-3, B-5, C, E, and Vitamin-K.

Minerals: Sodium, Calcium, Potassium, Magnesium, Zinc, Iron, Manganese, and Cooper.

Rich in Proteins and Amino Acids.

Shark Cartilage

Garlic: Garlic is mentioned in the Bible and the Talmud. Hippocrates, Galen, Pliny the Elder, and Discoredes all mention the use of garlic for many conditions, including parasites, respiratory problems, poor digestion, and low energy. Its use in China was first mentioned in A.D. 510. Louis Pasteur confirmed the antibacterial action of garlic in 1858. Human population studies show that eating garlic regularly reduces the risk of esophageal, stomach, and colon cancer. This is partly due to its ability to reduce the formation of carcinogenic compounds. Animal and test tube studies also show that garlic and its sulfur compounds inhibit the growth of different types of cancer, especially breast and skin tumors.

Alfa Alfa: This is a plant with abundant nutritive elements necessary in our daily diet. It is rich in Proteins, Vitamin A, B-1 (thiamine), B-2 (riboflavin), vitamin C, K, Phosphorus, Calcium, Zinc, Iron, Magnesium, Manganese, and Cooper.

Boldo: Scientists believe that boldine is responsible for the plant's choloretic (bile stimulating) and diuretic actions. In conjunction with other herbs, such as cascara, rhubarb, and gentian, boldo has been reported to improve symptoms related to loss of appetite.

It is thought that 60% of all degenerative diseases are directly related to a factor in our daily diet. Diet and Nutrition are probably the most important factor in the prevention of degenerative disease. Preven-CA is a natural product in capsule form, which delivers most of the nutrients that you regularly require and are not contained in your daily diet. Many of these nutrients are necessary for our body to work at its highest potential.

Daily Complete Liquid Multivitamin

Multiple vitamin/mineral (MVM) supplements contain a variable number of essential nutrients. Their primary purpose is to provide a convenient way to take a variety of supplemental nutrients from a single product, in order to prevent vitamin or mineral deficiencies, as well as to achieve higher intakes of nutrients believed to be of benefit above typical dietary levels. Both Dr. Philip Binzel and Dr. Ernsto Contreras have always included a multivitamin complex as part of their cancer protocol.

Daily Complete is a 100% plant sourced vegetarian liquid formula. One ounce provides you with 190 of the vitamins, minerals, antioxidants and important accessory nutrients that your body needs on a daily basis. This all-natural formula helps assure that you will obtain the nourishment you need while undergoing metabolic therapy. Daily Complete contains Phenalgin, which is one of the most powerful antioxidants on the planet.

Barley Grass (Just Barley Juice)

Barley Grass therapy consists primarily of detoxification and consuming as a drink several times each day. Fresh barley grass in this form is a potent source of many vitamins, minerals and plant enzymes. Thus, it is said to be nature's own nutritional program. Barley grass also contain Vitamin B17 (Amygdalin/Laetrile), although other sources, such as apricot seeds are more potent.

Barley grass juice is the powdered form of the pure natural juice of young barley leaves. It provides one of the widest spectrums of naturally occurring nutrients available in a single source on the earth today. Just Barley contains at least 16 vitamins, 23 minerals, 18 amino acids, and numerous usable enzymes. It also has one of the most alkaline pH factors available in a food and contains large amounts of natural chlorophyll (the blood of the plant).

Just Barley is grown from select organic seeds at over 5000 ft elevation in the mineral rich soil of an ancient volcanic lakebed. Just Barley is irrigated with pure mineral spring water and harvested at the peak of nutrition. It is processed "on sight" being dehydrated at 880 F to lock in nutritional potency.

Just Barley Green is also guaranteed to be pure, vegetarian, and 100% organically grown. It is also guaranteed to be 100% pure barley juice extract containing no binders, fillers, sweeteners, or additives of any kind.

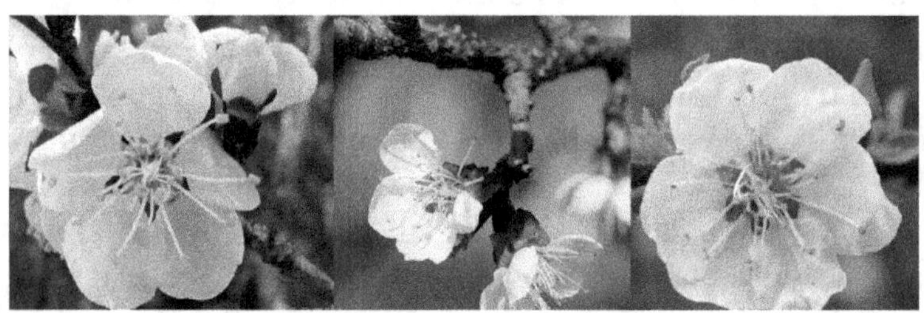

Accessory Metabolic Supplements

(Not routinely prescribed but recommended)

Maximol (Neways International)

The huge rise in incidences of cancer and other degenerative diseases are primarily due to the depleted vitamin/mineral content in today's western diet coupled with environmental/chemical toxin factors. The key nutritional ingredients invariably missing for cancer are 817 and the trace mineral selenium. A recent US study showed an overall drop of 50% in cancer deaths and a fall of 37% in new cancer cases, especially lung, bowel and prostate - among 1,300 volunteers taking supplements for four years.

Mineral supplementation is most effective in the ionised 'liquid suspension' form, assisted by fulvic acid, where a 98% assimilation by the body is expected, as against 48% for chelated minerals and 10-12% for metallic minerals. Our bodies use minerals as raw material. The body cannot manufacture these and so have to be present in the food and liquids we ingest. Sadly, as mentioned previously, our food chain is severely depleted of minerals, resulting in over 150 nutritional deficiency diseases that are now striking our societies with increasing intensity.

To combat this very real threat, mineral and vitamin supplementation is essential for everyone and can literally make the difference between life or death, especially for those with cancer. To combat this threat, Neways has formulated Maximol Solutions, probably the world's most complete liquid nutritional supplement, which contains 67 essential and trace minerals, 17 essential vitamins, 21 amino acids, three enzymes, and lactobacillus acidophilus. To provide greater absorption of all these ingredients, Maximol has been formulated with nature's natural chelator, used by plants and animals for the absorption of minerals and nutrients - organic fulvic acid. It is known that fulvic acid aids in the transport and assimilation of minerals and nutrients into living cells. This may in part be due to its low molecular weight, its electrical potential, and its bio-transporting ability. Fulvic acid aids in the selective trading or supply of minerals and other nutrient factors inside the cell. Fulvic acid is effective at neutralizing a wide range of toxic material - from heavy metals and radioactive waste to petrochemicals.

Before minerals can be utilized, they must first be converted from their particular colloidal state to a micro-colloidal state. Thus, for greater bioavailability, Neways has formulated Maximol Solutions as an organic fulvic acid complexed micro-colloidal solution. In this form, Maximol provides higher percentages of easily assimilated minerals than non-ionised colloidal mineral supplements, whose particles are often too large for easy absorption.

Revenol (Neways International)

Scientists tell us that vitamins A, C, and E, as well as beta carotene and other antioxidant bioflavonoids, are vitally important to good health. Antioxidants have about 20 times the power of Vitamin C and 50 times that of Vitamin E. The Neways product Revenol contains antioxidants that are broad-spectrum. Revenol contains antioxidants from maritime pine bark and grape seed pycnogenols extracts - up to 95% in concentration and bioavailability. Revenol also contains curcuminoids - nature's most powerful and aggressive antioxidant, which is around 150 times more powerful than Vitamin E, about 60 times more powerful than Vitamin C, and about 3 times more powerful than antioxidants from maritime pine bark and grape seed pycnogenols extract.

Revenol also contains ginkgo biloba for the brain and circulatory system; alpha and beta carotene to increase potency; Esterfied Vitamin C - a bonded form of Vitamin C that increases its power and residual retention in the body (up to 3 days); natural Vitamin E for greater absorption and effectiveness. Micro-spheres are also included which bond to the intestinal wall, allowing up to 400% more of the ingredients to be digested and absorbed.

Each tablet of Revenol supplies over 60 milligrams of curcuminoids and maritime pine bark and grape seed extract. An independent study on antioxidants has been conducted by Russian biochemists. As they announce their findings to the World Health Organization, Revenol is expected to be listed as the world's Number 1 effective antioxidant.

Cascading Revenol

Neways has also released an exciting, further version of Revenol, named Cascading Revenol. Free radicals, unpaired oxygen molecules that are hungry to scavenge additional oxygen, damage healthy cells and are especially dangerous for cancer suffers. Antioxidants such as Vitamin C neutralise the damage caused by these free radicals. The problem is, after having entered the body, most antioxidant molecular structures will grab one free radical and then change into an inert state, ceasing to be of further scavenging value. The additional problem is that even when an antioxidant neutralizes a free radical, the process creates an off-shoot free radical that is slightly different and less potent in variety, which in turn creates another, and so on. Typical antioxidants have no ability to address this free radical cascading effect.

However Cascading Revenol's technologically advanced formulation actually regenerates these scavenging molecules so that they can neutralise multiple free radicals. So, instead of only one free radical being destroyed per antioxidant molecule, each molecule is able to change structure and repeat the process again and again. Thus the value of each individual antioxidant molecule increases exponentially. Cascading Revenol's unique action is devastating to the free radical onslaught that damages cancer sufferers. This product can be an essential component in any B17 Metabolic Therapy treatment.

Cassie-Tea (Neways International)

Cassie-Tea is a traditional health formula designed to help assist the body's efforts to eliminate toxins that accumulate in the body with age. Turkey rhubarb root supports liver and intestinal health, while sheep sorrel herb and burdock root help in the body's efforts to maintain the blood stream. Slippery Elm helps soothe irritated mucus membranes and soothe and moisten the respiratory tract.

Neways' Cassie-Tea is the same as the famous Essiac. René Caisse, a Canadian nurse, treated thousands of cancer patients for sixty years using an herbal drink popular with the Ojibway Indians. In 1937 the Royal Cancer Commission of Canada conducted hearings concerning Essiac ('Caisse' backwards) and pronounced as its conclusion that the preparation had marked anti-cancer properties. Tom Mower, the president of Neways, obtained the formulation for Cassie-Tea from a source that used to mix the tea for Nurse Caisse. Cassie-Tea is an excellent nutritional supplement for those undergoing B17 Metabolic Therapy.

Hawaiian Noni Juice (Neways International)

The fruit juice of Morinda citrifolia contains a polysaccharide-rich substance with marked anti-tumor activity, according to recent studies into the famous fruit. This research, performed at the University of Hawaii, has resulted in exciting new and scientifically reputable evidence for the potential benefits of Noni fruit juice in the treatment of cancer. Neways Authentic Hawaiian Noni features all the health-enhancing benefits of the noni plant as well as raspberry and blueberry extracts - both powerful antioxidants.

Purge / Feelin' Good (Neways International)

Researchers state that the majority of people especially those with cancer, play host to one form of parasite or another. Parasites are life forms that are uninvited lodgers in our bodies who do not pay rent. They can range from tiny amoebae detectable only with a microscope to tapeworms many feet in length.

We inadvertently pick up parasites through our day-to-day activities and especially through eating undercooked or contaminated food. Blood flukes for instance can enter our systems through infected drinking water and take up residence in the bladder, intestines, liver, lungs, rectum and spleen, laying their eggs and breeding in humans for up to 20 years. Trichina worm larvae found in undercooked pork migrate from the intestines through the blood and lymphatic system, eventually lodging in muscles. Threadworm larvae enter skin from the soil and pass through the bloodstream to the lungs, sometimes causing pneumonia.

Eliminating parasites is effectively a three-phase program. Killing them, flushing them out and then supplementing our relieved bodies with healthy nutrients to maintain optimum health. Neways features this very effective three-phase program, employing their products Purge, Feelin' Good and Maximol Solutions respectively to execute the clean-up, leaving you bug-free and, most importantly, invigorated and strengthened to avoid re-infestation.

Dimethyl sulfoxide (DMSO)

DMSO is a by-product of the wood and paper industry and has gained prominence in recent times as a highly effective agent in the treatment of herpes, cancer and other diseases. It is known for its ability to permeate living tissue and stimulate cellular processes. Dr. Morton Walker in his book, DMSO: The New Healing Power, describes how it blocks pain, reduces inflammation, kills bacteria and funguses, reduces blood clotting, improves circulation, neutralises free radicals, stimulates the immune system, and hastens the healing of wounds. It is used for everything from minor cuts and cold sores to insect bites, athletic injuries, arthritic aches and pains, and cancer.

DMSO is known for its unique ability solvent that penetrates the blood/brain barrier and is used with B17 intravenously to deliver the principal treatment deep into the body without changing the latter's chemical structure. DMSO is renowned for its ability to penetrate the body's tissue rapidly and completely. Some clinics use it on all types of cancer, though doctors prefer not to use it with cases of liver or kidney disease.

The dose most doctors use is as follows:

Intravenous Use: 3 cc to 5 cc of DMSO for every 10cc of Vitamin B-17 in a 30 cc syringe. e.g. Each 3 gram vial of vitamin B-17 contains 10 cc. The contents of two 3 gram vials would be mixed with 6 to 10cc of DMSO, in a 30 cc syringe.

Topical Use: Doctors have patients mix 1.4 oz (42cc) of DMSO with 0.6 oz (18cc) of pure water in a glass bottle (not plastic); Using natural cotton (not synthetic), 1 teaspoon of this mix is applied 2 or 3 times per day to a soft skin area of the body, leaving on for 10 minutes and then rinsing area. DMSO may be applied close to the affected area. Most people feel that its garlic-like odor is a small price to pay for its unique benefits.

Diet

The diet can be summarized as follows: If it is animal or if it comes from animal, you cannot have it. If it is not animal or does not come from animal, you can have it, but you cannot cook it. Patient should take away all meat, all poultry, all fish, all eggs, cheese, cottage cheese and milk.

The reason for such a diet is that Dr. Krebs et al. had found that the cancer cell had a protein lining (or covering), and that if the body dissolves that protein lining, it would kill the cancer cell. The dissolving of that protein lining, they said, is done by the enzymes trypsin and chymotrypsin, which are secreted by the pancreas. It is important to understand that it takes large quantities of trypsin and chymotrypsin to digest animal protein. Thus, the cancer patient who is eating animal protein may be using up all, or almost all, of his trypsin and chymotrypsin for digestive purposes. This leaves none of these enzymes available to the rest of the body.

The patient would be on this diet for a minimum of four months. In that period of time, I was attempting to free the trypsin and the chymotrypsin from being used up for digestive purposes and to put these enzymes back into the body in order to restore the body's first line of defense against cancer.

The reason for the fresh fruits and fresh vegetables is, again, because of enzymes. There are some enzymes in fresh fruits and vegetables which are tremendously important in good nutrition. Any temperature over 130 degrees will destroy the enzymes in the fruits and vegetables. For this reason, the fruits and vegetables may not be cooked, canned or bottled. Frozen foods from the grocery store are also prohibited because most of these frozen foods have been processed in some manner. They have either been blanched, pasteurized or sterilized so that the enzymes have been destroyed. Those who do their own home freezing are permitted to do so as long as they do not blanch the foods before they are frozen.

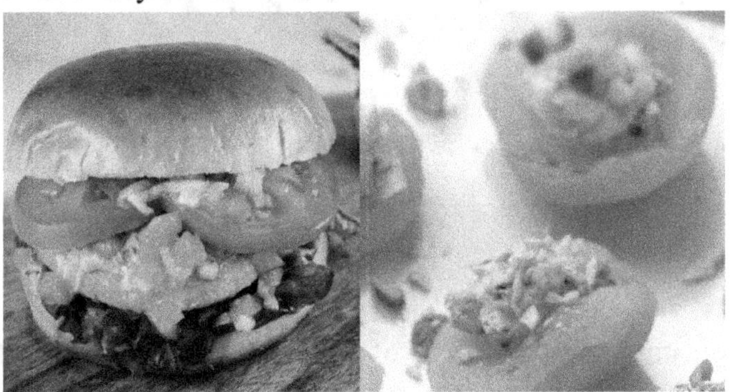

This means a diet that is high in salads. Salad dressings are permitted as long as the salad dressings do not contain anything which the patient may not have. Salad dressings which contain egg or sugar are not permitted. Patients should make their own salad dressings. This is fine as long as they start with a pure vegetable oil and use no refined sugar. Do not attempt to severely limit the salt intake unless you have a medical problem which requires it. Salt may be used in moderation, but any salt that is used should be sea salt. The mineral content of sea salt is far superior to mineral content of the salt we normally use. Iodized sea salt is fine, if they need it. Use a variety of other herbs and spices in order to vary the salad dressings so you are not eating the same thing over and over again.

The patients are not permitted anything which contains white flour or white sugar. Whole wheat flour can be used instead of white flour. In the place of sugar they can use either honey or molasses. Foods containing preservatives are kept to an absolute minimum.

The patients are encouraged to have as wide a variety of vegetables as possible. All vegetables are somewhat similar, but each vegetable, in its own way, supplies something nutrition-wise that no other vegetable has. So try to consume at least some of every vegetable available at that season, within any two-week period of time.

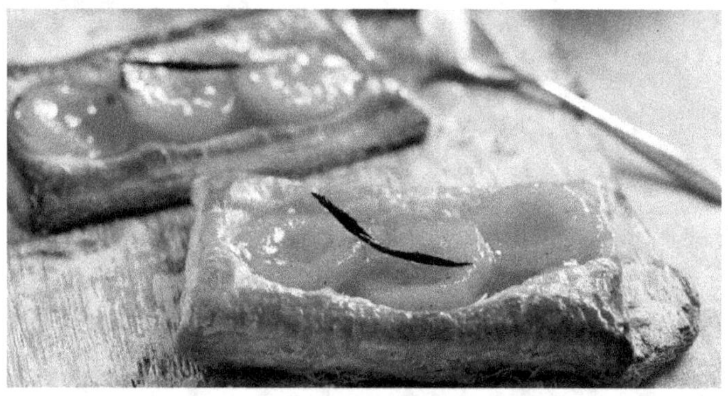

Consume wide a variety of fruits as possible, except for the citrus fruits. Oranges, lemons, grapefruit and tomatoes (Yes, tomatoes are a citrus fruit.) are not to be more than ten percent of their fruit intake. Other fruits such as apples, peaches, and pears contain far more nutrition than do the citrus fruits. Except for the citrus fruits, you should eat the seeds of your fruits. Apple seeds, grape seeds, apricot kernels, peach kernels, etc. have a high nitriloside content.

With the combined fruits and vegetables, patients should have about sixty percent vegetables and about forty percent fruits. Do not weigh and measure your fruits and vegetables, but you keep the vegetable intake a little higher than the fruit intake.

Protein in the diet is, of course, very necessary. However, rather than using animal protein, use vegetable protein. Vegetable protein requires nothing in the way of the enzymes trypsin and chymotrypsin for digestion. The things that you use for your protein content can be cooked. You do not alter or harm a vegetable protein by cooking it.

Whole Grains

It is important that the patients read the ingredients on the labels of everything they buy. Everything labeled "Whole Wheat Bread" is not necessarily whole grain. Many of these breads contain only a small amount of whole grain and contain a large amount of white flour, white sugar and preservatives.

Whole grain cereals are permissible as long as they do not contain sugar. Most of these do contain some preservatives, but the amount is usually quite small. Do not use some low fat milk or skim milk on your cereal. Whole wheat macaroni, noodles, spaghetti, etc. are also readily available and are good sources of protein.

Corn

This is an excellent source of protein. You may have corn-on-the-cob (which may be cooked), pop corn and corn meal in any form. Corn meal mush, grits and cornbread are permitted. It is necessary, in order to make cornbread, to use some egg and some milk. This is not a problem because the amounts of the egg and milk are quite small.

Buckwheat

This is high in protein. Buckwheat pancakes and pure maple syrup are excellent. Again, in order to make the buckwheat pancakes, you must use a little egg and milk. This is not a sufficient amount to cause a problem.

Butter

Butter in small amounts is permitted. Any butter that is used should be real butter rather than any margarine. Vegetable oil hardened (containing Trans fats) into a solid is detrimental to good nutrition.

Nuts

These are an excellent source of protein. These includes all nuts except the peanut. Roasted peanuts are not permitted because of an acid that is formed in the roasting. This is not true of any other nuts. Raw peanuts are permitted, but not roasted peanuts.

Dried Fruits

Dried fruits, such as dates, raisins, and figs, are excellent nutrition and provide protein.

Beans

Some vegetables, such as those in the bean family and in the brown rice family, cannot be eaten raw. Soup beans, lentils, spit-pea, navy beans and kidney beans, are an excellent source of protein and should be an important part of this diet. Meals like bean soup and cornbread provide a complete protein, as would a meal of beans and brown rice.

You should emphasize, again, the necessity of eating raw fruits and raw vegetables. Everything that can be eaten raw should be eaten raw. So many of the things you cook can be eaten raw. For example, broccoli, spinach, turnips, potatoes, and green beans can all be eaten raw.

Beverages

No milk, other than that used on cereal and in cooking, is permitted. No caffeine is permitted. This means no coffee, no Sanka, no Decaf, etc. Natural coffee substitutes are permitted along with any of the herb teas.

Follow this type of program for at least four months. Dr. Philip E. Binzel, Jr., M.D., in twenty years of work in this field, experienced that it takes that long to get this defense mechanism to function normally. If, at the end of the first four months, the patient is not doing very well, continue the strict diet for as long as necessary. At the end of four months, if the patient is doing well, then liberalize the diet. Then allow the patient to add chicken, turkey and fish to his diet. Ninety percent of the diet at that time consists of the original strict diet plus the chicken, turkey and fish. The other ten percent of the diet may include red meats, cooked vegetables and dairy products. Remember that, within any two-weeks period of time, the red meats, cooked vegetables and dairy products should never exceed more than ten percent of your total diet.

The patients are told that they also must stay on their vitamins, enzymes and Laetrile until the age of 130. Please call me on your 130th birthday (although I am not sure what my address will be at that time), and we will discuss the possibility of reducing the dosage of some of these. *This is simply my way of emphasizing to the patient the fact that you don't cure cancer. You can control it as long as the defense mechanisms continue to function normally. If a patient goes back to his old eating habits, he will soon be back in trouble again.*

Facts to Know About Laetrile …

Dr. Antonio Jimenez says laetrile has several positive effects, including direct anticancer activity, analgesic properties, and well-being enhancement. He describes Laetrile Therapy as a safe, productive part of an integrative cancer treatment program.

Laetrile is banned in the U.S., but it is administered legally in several clinics in Mexico, Germany, and parts of Asia, usually intravenously in high doses. Apricot seeds and apricot-based pills can be purchased in the U.S. and taken as a nutritional supplement. (Alive And Well)

Frequently Asked Questions

1) Q. What is Laetrile (vitamin B-17/Amygdalin)?

Laetrile, commonly known as Vitamin B-17 or Amygdalin, is a natural chemotherapeutic agent found in over 1,200 plants, particularly in the seeds of common fruits such as apricots, peaches, plums, and apples. It is a diglucocide with a cyanide radical that is highly "bio-accessible." This means that it penetrates through the cellular membrane reaching high intra-cellular concentrations easily.

2) Q. Where can I purchase vitamin B-17 (Laetrile)?

You may take Laetrile Therapy at OASIS of Hope Hospital in Fracc. Playas de Tijuana, Terrazas, 22504 Tijuana, Baja California, Mexico, you may visit them on the web at http://www.oasisofhope.com or Phone +52 664 631 6100. The Oasis of Hope Hospital is providing Laetrile Therapy and other alternative cancer treatments to its customers. The clinic was founded by the physician, Dr. Ernsto Contreras. This is one of the best center for alternative cancer treatments including Laetrile treatment.

You may obtain vitamin B-17 (Laetrile) and most of the metabolic products mentioned on

http://www.cytopharmaonline.com,

http://www.healthgenesis.com

and through vitamin and supplement companies throughout the world. Do some research on Google before you buy the products. If you live in the U.S., it will not be possible for you to obtain vitamin B17 due to recent FDA bans and customs restrictions, but you can buy vitamin B17 online.

3) Q. Why is Laetrile "illegal" or "banned" in the United States?

There is no federal law against Laetrile, nor does Laetrile appear on an official list of proscribed items. The State of California has specific laws against the use of Laetrile for human cancer, as long as cancer is defined as a "space-occupying new growth" or neoplasm. A number of other states make the use of Laetrile in cancer indirectly "illegal" by giving cancer advisory committees the power to regulate the use of any remedies, proven or unproven. The Food and Drug Administration has used regulations, not law, to ban the interstate shipment and sale of Laetrile by alleging that it is either an "unlicensed new "drug" or an "unsafe or adulterated food or food additive." Though it is neither, the de facto (but certainly not de jure) "illegalization" of Laetrile springs from the FDA's regulatory ban, the specific California laws, and the pressure brought against physicians by state boards of medical examiners which control the licensing of such physicians. It is virtually as inappropriate to call Laetrile or vitamin B-17 illegal as it is to construe vitamin C, or niacin as illegal. In California, despite the specific laws, the right of doctors to use vitamin B-17 as metabolic therapy, and without making specific claims as to "curing cancer," was established by court decisions in a number of cases.

At the Mexican border, U.S. Customs has permitted the entry of amygdalin for private use without benefit of even an affidavit for over a decade. Amygdalin is an extract of apricot kernels, which makes it a food supplement and nothing more. Under FDA guidelines, however, any substance that is used to treat a disorder can be classified a drug. In the U.S., it appears as though the FDA has the authority to label ANYTHING a "new drug" when a claim is made for that substance or even suggestions given as to how to take it.

As of 2000, there are different State Statutes in the U.S. that make the possession and use of Laetrile perfectly legal in some states and illegal in others. The FDA, however, has banned the commercialization of Laetrile in the U.S. by making it illegal to import it for resale, or to transport it from State to State. Therefore, If you are in the U.S., you will not be able to purchase Laetrile.

4) Q. What is the recommended daily dosage of vitamin B-17 for prevention?

While exact amounts of B-17 for a "minimum daily requirement" in cancer surveillance have not been established, the basic concept is that sufficient daily B-17 may be obtained by following either of two suggestions:

One, according to Dr. Krebs, eating all the B-17-containing fruits whole (seeds included), but not eating more of the seeds by themselves than you would be eating if you ate them in the whole fruit. Example: if you eat three apples a day, the seeds in the three apples are sufficient B-17. You would not eat a pound of apple seeds.

Second, one peach or apricot kernel per 10 lbs. of body weight is believed to be more than sufficient as a normal safeguard in cancer prevention, although precise numbers may vary from person to person in accordance with individual metabolism and dietary habits. A 170-lb man, for example, might consume 17 apricot or peach kernels per day and receive a biologically reasonable amount of vitamin B-17. Two or three Vitamin B17 tablets (100 mg) is an acceptable supplemental dosage per day.

And two important notes: Certainly, you can consume too much of anything. Too many kernels or seeds, for example, can be expected to produce unpleasant side effects. These natural foods should be consumed in biologically rational amounts (no more than 30 to 35 kernels per day).

5) Q. What is the difference between apricot seeds and B-17 100 mg tablets when used for prevention? Is one better than the other? Do I need to take both?

Dr. Krebs always suggested that the raw form of vitamin B-17 (e.g. apricot kernels) is better than the purified form when used for prevention. This holds true for any other food: The raw form of vitamin C (e.g. grapefruits and oranges), for example, is also better than the pill. The difference between these two forms of vitamin B-17 is that the tablet is a more convenient method of administration; the seeds have a bitter taste to them and some people prefer the convenience of a tablet. Some people have dentures and simply find it difficult to chew on the seeds. Most people take both. It is completely safe to take both forms as many cancer patients take up to 4 times the amount of seeds recommended for a non-cancer sufferer, and up to 50 times more of the purified form (tablet form). It is not necessary to take both forms but, as stated above, you can get away with doing so while getting a reasonable amount of vitamin B-17.

IMPORTANT: Cancer patients, however, may require higher, more purified forms of vitamin B-17. It would be impossible to get the amount of vitamin B-17 needed to control existing cancer from the seeds alone. One would have to eat way too many seeds and this may, of course, produce unpleasant side effects.

6) Q. I have been diagnosed with Cancer. Will vitamin B-17 work on any type of cancer?

Dr. Krebs says "yes". Cancer cells all have the exact same characteristics. Cancer cells, no matter the type of cancer, are known as Trophoblast. These cells contain an enzyme called Beta-glucosidase, also known as the unlocking enzyme. When Laetrile comes in contact with the enzyme beta-glucosidase, the Laetrile is broken down to form two molecules of glucose, one molecule of benzaldehyde and one molecule of hydrogen cyanide (HCN). Within the body, the cancer cell-and only the cancer cell-contains that enzyme. The key word here is that the HCN must be FORMED. It is not floating around freely in the Laetrile and then released. It must be manufactured. The enzyme beta-glucosidase, and only that enzyme, is capable of manufacturing the HCN from Laetrile thereby affecting the cancer cell-and only the cancer cell.

If there are no cancer cells in the body, there is no beta-glucosidase. If there is no beta-glucosidase, no HCN will be formed from the Laetrile.

7) Q. I have been diagnosed with Cancer. What should be my dosage of vitamin B-17, what do I take it with, and how long do I take it for?

"If you have Cancer, the most important single consideration is to get the maximum amount of Vitamin B17 into your body in the shortest period of time. This is secondary to the medical skill involved in administering it, which is relatively minimal." - Ernst T. Krebs, Jr.

Many people take vitamin B-17 and B-17 only, and many people order it as part a whole complete combined metabolic protocol. The ideal thing to do is to always make vitamin B-17 part of a multi-faceted program incorporating numerous related elements, each of which plays an important role in the success of the complete therapy (See Metabolic Therapies).

But for the purpose of answering the question the dosages recommended by Dr. Contreras of the Oasis of Hope Hospital should be as follows:

Initial Phase (Phase I): AMYGDALIN (Vitamin B17) 6 grams, intravenous (Most Effective Method), once a day, for 21 days. (2 vials directly into any vein or catheter) - See protocols.

Or: AMYGDALIN 3 grams (six 500mg tablets), orally, per day, for 21 days (See protocols). Along with Laetrile, the OASIS Hospital utilizes pancreatic enzymes (proteolytic enzymes), Vitamin C, Pangamic Acid (B15), AHCC (active Hexose Correlated Compound), Shark Cartilage (100% pure), vitamin A (Emulsified), Barley Grass, antioxidants, and other nutrients (see Metabolic Therapy Components). The idea is to help the body fight the cancer very aggressively, without doing any harm to the patient, while strengthening the immune system.

Subsequent Phase (Phase II):

AMYGDALIN (Vitamin B17) 2 grams (Four 500mg tablets), orally, per day, for the following three months, along with all the components of Phase II Metabolic Therapy (see protocols).

After Phase II: Phase III Metabolic Therapy consists of either a continuation of Phase II or maintenance program if the cancer is in remission (See Maintenance of Remission).

Vitamin B17 is water soluble and non-toxic. It is as safe as sugar or water and safer than aspirin. A small percentage of people feel nauseous when taking high doses of it at one time. This is also common when taking too much sugar, salt, or water at one time. If this is the case take less amounts of the vitamin B17 tablets more often throughout the day. If you presently have cancer, you can take between 6 to 10 of the 500 milligram tablets per day for the first 21 to 30 days. If you find that you are getting nauseous, cut the tablets in half and have one every waking hour. It might be a good idea to have some food in your stomach just before taking the vitamin. After the initial 21-30 days of this amount of vitamin B17 a subsequent dose of 4 to 6 tablets per day for the following three months is the proper protocol (See Phase I and II Metabolic Therapies).

8) Q. Is it necessary to have the seeds and the Vitamin together when undergoing metabolic therapy?

Dr. Contreras says "yes". Certain components of the seeds are not included in the purified forms of amygdalin. The seeds are the raw form of vitamin B-17, containing many other nutrients that act synergistically with the purified form to help its active ingredients assimilate into the body. To start, it is recommended that along with the purified forms of B-17, either intravenous or oral, cancer patients eat one apricot seed for every 10 lbs of body weight. If this dosage is tolerated well, it may be increased to 30 to 35 kernels per day. IMPORTANT: For adults, more than 6 per hour or 30 per day is not recommended.

It is important to emphasize that it is a good idea to have some food in the stomach when taking high doses of B-17 (including the seeds). When eating the seeds, it is also important to eat considerable amount of Nitrilosidic fruits. Such fruits are those which carry these types of (e.g. Apricots, peaches, plums, nectarines, apples, pears, cherries). There is something in the flesh of the fruit, which will neutralise the minute traces of beta-glucosidase present in saliva, stomach, and the intestines, which is what may cause some people to feel nauseous.

9) Q. Are apricot seeds made available in the pit or out of the pit? Do we have to break the pits open to extract the kernel?

Most companies make available bags of fresh whole apricot kernels out of the pit and ready to eat. See Metabolic Therapy Components for more detailed information about Apricot kernels. For sources of apricot kernels see Contacts.

10) Q. What should I take along with Vitamin B-17?

If you have cancer it is recommended by Dr. Contreras (One of the Pioneers of B17 treatment and medical director at the OASIS of Hope Hospital) that you undergo a therapy that will equip your immune system to fight against cancer. Their special detoxification program will create what is necessary to get the best results. Along with Laetrile, the Contreras team uses pancreatic enzymes, Vitamin C, Shark Cartilage (100% pure), vitamin A (emulsified), pangamic acid (vitamin B-15), antioxidants, nitrilosidic foods (apricot kernels) and other nutrients (see Protocols). Every one of these nutrients plays an important role in the success of the complete therapy. Pancreatic enzymes, for example, occur naturally in pineapple and papaya among other foods. They are also produced by our pancreas and aid in the digestion of animal protein. Their job is to help burn away the negative protein coating that surrounds and protects the cancer cell making it vulnerable to your immune system.

The purpose of metabolic therapy is mainly to restore wellness. Unfortunately, by the time most cancer patients seek alternative medicine their bodies have suffered extensive damage due to the effects of chemotherapy, radiation, surgery, or the cancer itself. Because of this, other nutrients should be considered to help significantly in restoring wellness. Joint Fuel, Bone Meal, and Bovine cartilage may help build up the bones again if you have had bone cancer. Maitake and Shittake mushrooms (the most scientifically studied mushrooms) have been found to have an antiviral substance called lentinan, which stimulates the body's immune system and deactivates viruses. Other nutrients which have been extensively researched for cancer therapy include the ESSIAC Formula, AHCC, coenzyme Q10, grape seed extract, cat's claw, IP-6, colloidal minerals, vitamin E, Ginger, Beta Carotene, Multivitamin/minerals, Antioxidants, Hydrazine sulphate, echinacea, milk thistle, melatonin, noni, and raw thymus, most of which are available through vitamin companies. It is common knowledge among scientists and holistic doctors that combinations of therapies are more effective than just one. You may customize your metabolic treatment based on your specific needs (See Metabolic Therapy Components for specific information on metabolic products).

11) Q. How can I get the intravenous form of B-17 administered?

Any nurse or doctor can simply make a house visit and administer this form of B-17. It is completely safe and non-toxic and does not produce any side effects. You can simply ask a nurse or doctor friend or relative who is willing to give you the injections to do it. It is important that you find someone who agrees to give you the injections before you purchase this form of B-17. Some sources of B17 may not issue credits or refunds on injectable formulas or specially imported products. If you would like information on the OASIS of Hope Hospital in Fracc. Playas de Tijuana, Terrazas, 22504 Tijuana, Baja California, Mexico), you may visit them on the web at http://www.oasisofhope.com or Phone +52 664 631 6100.

The best effects from Laetrile use seem to be when it is used as part of a bask nutritional or metabolic therapy which also involves the administration of other vitamins, certain enzymes, and a diet from which animal protein has been mostly removed (See OASIS Phase I and II Metabolic Therapies).

12) Q. Are there any risks in getting the injectable form of vitamin B-17 administered? I am a qualified medical professional, what is my risk in administering it to a loved one?

The question should be "what is the risk in not getting it administered?", or, "what is the risk of not giving it to my loved one?". This form of vitamin B-17 is not only safe and non-toxic. Sugar or water are more toxic. On the contrary, a majority of Laetrile-treated patients report positive responses, ranging from an increase in the feeling of well-being and even a brighter outlook on life, to such noticeable reactions as an increase in appetite, weight gain and, frequently, restoration of natural color, reduction or elimination of cancer-connected pain and of cancer-caused fetor.

13) Q. Can I Take Vitamin B17 with chemotherapy or radiation, or if I am scheduled for surgery?

Metabolic physicians agree that under the above orthodox treatments metabolic therapy is not only recommended but also absolutely necessary. Orthodox doctors use chemotherapy, radiation, and surgery in an effort to get to the cancer while often times causing severe damage to the body's organs and defense mechanisms (see The 4 Optional Modes of Cancer Therapy). Cancer, by definition, is a Chronic Metabolic disease and must be treated as such. The word "chronic" means that once it manifests, it will continue to remain uncontrolled and uncorrected if it does not get taken care of. "Metabolic" simply means that the only way to take care of it is with factors, water- and oil-soluble, normal to the diet. The problem with orthodox treatments is that they do not target the underlying cause of the problem but its symptom. Metabolic therapy, on the other hand, targets the nutritional deficiency factor that keeps the body from fighting the cancer while strengthening the immune system.

Ideally, you should ask your doctor what their success rate is with chemotherapy, radiation, and/or surgery for your specific type of cancer. Ask him to give you true statistics. You may even ask him to show you the description of the drugs you are about to become exposed to in a PDR (Physician's Desk Reference). It is important to know beforehand whether these treatments will actually help you or hurt you. *In some cases, though, the treatment becomes worse than the disease itself. **If you are about to have surgery, or even a biopsy, where the cancer cells are going to be disturbed, it is imperative that you take vitamin B-17 to kill the remaining free cells (see The Truth About Surgeries and Biopsies). Vitamin B-17 can only help and will definitely not hurt.

*Clinical Oncology for Medical Students and Physicians, op. cit, pp.32 , 34

*Spontaneous Regression of Cancer: The Metabolic Triumph of the Host!", op. cit.,pp. 136, 137.

14) Q. I have undergone chemotherapy, radiation, and surgery. Can vitamin B-17 still help me?

Dr. Krebs says "yes", but remember this: Vitamin B-17 metabolic therapy will go into the body to help your immune system fight the cancer without doing any harm to you. What it may not do, is correct the irreparable damage sometimes caused by excessive chemotherapy or radiation, or by the cancer itself. According to Dr. Krebs, anyone at any stage is a candidate for metabolic treatment.

15) Q. How long does it take to see results? How long will it take to rid my body of cancer?

There are two kinds of results that are usually observed while undergoing Laetrile Metabolic Therapy. These can be classified as both subjective and objective:

Subjective results are usually seen immediately after beginning treatment: These include decrease of pain, indicated by a decrease in the amount or frequency of the use of narcotics or sedatives, increase in the sense of well-being, increased appetite, disappearance of fetor from lesions, increased energy or endurance, increase in weight, and increase in muscle strength.

Objective results include improvement in blood and urine chemistry, increased tissue repair, decrease of tumefaction, decrease in the output of presumptive chorionic gonadotrophin in the serum or urine, and total regression of all symptoms of the disease. Objective results can take between 3 weeks to 4 months to manifest. The time needed to develop the maximum response is four months to over a year.

"Overall, the cancer cells become affected immediately", says Dr. Krebs, "In certain cases, as with bone and brain cancer, it takes a little longer for the vitamin to absorb deep into the body" (see Notes on the Behavior of Tumors Under Vitamin B17 Therapy). According to Dr. Krebs skin cancers react the quickest: "Within one week a noticeable difference is seen and in many cases complete regression of all symptoms is achieved in less than three weeks. Carcinomas can take a few months to shrink, and, in some cases, cervical cancer has been noted to completely regress in less than three weeks."

16) Q. I am a cancer survivor; what is the recommended maintenance dose of vitamin B-17?

According to Dr. Krebs, a severe cancer crisis brought under control may be maintained in a quiescent state by the oral administration of 1 gram (1000 mg) of Vitamin B-17 daily. However some patients claim to feel better or safer with a 1.5 to 2.0 grams of B-17 daily. Such dosage is determined by the patient's sense of well being, gain in strength, increased appetite, weight gain, and psychological improvement with reduction of anxiety and nervousness, with exhibition of a more nearly normal degree of optimism and interest in his environment.

Abnormal situations, stress or ill health of any kind have been known to be followed by a renewed outbreak or progression of the cancer process in some patients. Patients in whom the cancer is under control should be aware of these possibilities. When a cancer crisis has been successfully controlled for more than two years, with patient showing good objective responses in weight gain, increased strength, return to a more nearly normal state of activity and vigor, with negative CGH urine tests, and with an improvement in x-rays or other objective evidence, the maintenance dose may be reduced to dietary levels of nitriloside of at least 500 milligrams of Vitamin B-17 per day.

17) Q. What is the success rate with my specific type of cancer?

Success rates for specific types of cancer are determined based on the stage of the cancer and/or the possible damage caused by the effects of chemotherapy, radiation, surgery, or the cancer itself. Vitamin B-17 can only help you and not hurt you. If you have just been diagnosed the ideal thing to do is to start metabolic therapy immediately. Dr. Krebs claimed a 98% success rate with Virgin cases (Primary cancers, non metastatic, where the patient has not had chemotherapy, radiation, or surgery). In cases where the patient has been exposed to chemotherapy, radiation, and/or surgery, it depends on how far the cancer has spread and what damage has been caused to the body by these treatments. In either case it is imperative to start vitamin therapy in order to correct the nutritional deficiency factor that allowed the disease to take over.

In conclusion, if you are able to eat, hold food down, urinate and defecate properly, you are coherent, and your bodily functions are normal, you are a perfect candidate for metabolic therapy.

18) Q. Why don't medical doctors use vitamin B17?

The answer to this question goes far beyond what we could possibly answer in this small section. Mr. G Edward Griffin has dedicated the entire second part of his book to "The Politics of Cancer Therapy", which shows with great detail examples of dishonesty and corruption in the field of drug research; a close look at the first major study which declared Laetrile (vitamin B17) "of no value;" proof that the study was fraudulent; the FDA's ruling against the use of Laetrile because it had not been tested; and the refusal then to allow anyone (except its opponents) to test it.

He also makes available an audio cassette titled "The Politics of Cancer Therapy", a review of the science of cancer therapy; a summary of the politics of cancer therapy; the early history of the I.G. Farben chemical and pharmaceutical cartel; the cartel's early success in the United States; and its "marriage" with DuPont, Standard Oil, and Ford. The drug cartel's influence over the nation's medical schools; the drug-oriented training given to all medical students; and the use of philanthropic foundations to obtain control over educational institutions. You may obtain this audiocassette from Mr. Griffin at http://www.realityzone.com

In conclusion, most doctors are obligated to use only those treatments that they're allowed to administer, even if they are not successful. Most doctors are not trained on how to prescribe "nutrition" as a way to treat disease. They only learn to treat the "symptom" while leaving the underlying cause of the problem uncontrolled and uncorrected. To fully educate yourself, start with Mr. Griffin's book "World Without Cancer". It can be bought on the Internet at http://www.realityzone.com. This book is one of a few that tell the true story of vitamin B17 and will guide you into further research that proves the simple answer to cancer 100%.

19) Q. The fact that cancer is a metabolic disease, what role does pollution have in that process?

Pollutants harm the liver and the liver is a great detoxifying organ of the body. If the liver is detoxifying an excess of estrogen, for example, and capacity of the liver is impaired by pollutants, the estrogen levels then may reach a concentration sufficient to induce cancer. When eating apples that have been sprayed with arsenic and we eat enough of these apples; the arsenic may produce hepatic cirrhosis, which may impair the capacity of the liver to detoxify certain carcinogens and thereby contribute to the development of cancer. If we are receiving a very high concentrating of Vitamin B17 this will offset the possibility of developing cancer, but these pollutants still can kill us by producing cirrhosis of the liver and destroying other vital cells.

20) Q. Is Vitamin B17 helpful against the devastating effects of excessive quantities of environmental or medical radiation?

No, and the reason for it is common sense. Throughout history the presence of radiation in such high concentrations was never anticipated. The organism may be beset with such onslaught and there are no mechanisms including Vitamin B-17, which can reverse the deadly effects of such excess radiation. These are some of the most devastating assaults that living tissues can sustain because not only do they affect the individual of one generation, but they may cripple, if not extinguish the immortal germ plasma, on which the continuity of the species itself relies.

21) Q. If we are supposed to eat seeds, why aren't we supplied with teeth for breaking through the pits?

There are societies that have not become too corrupted by the sophistication of modern technology. These people are capable of biting through the pit. We have even seen dogs break the pit and eat the seeds. Squirrels, chipmunks, bears, and higher primates such as monkeys ordinarily do it. Curators of zoos tell us when monkeys and apes are thrown fresh apricots, peaches and plums, in time, if they are thrown enough of them, they cease eating the sweet sugary fruit and they begin hoarding the pits. They manage to break open those pits. Primates will take them in hand and hammer them against a piece of concrete. Eating these seeds is universal among the nomads and among the higher animals.

22) Q. How do you keep the seeds once they are out of the pit?

You may keep the seeds indefinitely if you keep them sealed and under refrigeration. If you don't keep them under refrigeration the Vitamin B17 won't deteriorate, but the unsaturated fatty acids will turn rancid spoiling the seeds after a few months.

23) Q. Would there be a problem with the other drugs I am taking for pre-existing conditions (Diabetes, high cholesterol, ulcer, high blood pressure, etc)? I am currently taking: Lipitor, Glynase, Ranitidine, and occasionally Tylenol 3.

Metabolic physicians agree that cancer is a local manifestation of a systemic or metabolic disease. This means that some of those pre-existing conditions may have contributed to the formation of your malignancy. Metabolic therapy is meant to treat the entire body, not just the disease.

The answer to the question is yes, you can undergo metabolic therapy without it interfering with any of the drugs you are currently on. There is no substance yet known that can cause an adverse reaction with Laetrile. Remember, Laetrile is not a drug but a vitamin or food supplement.

The idea is to get metabolic therapy to make you well enough so that you do not have to depend on those medications for the rest of your life.

24) Q. I wonder though, are there documented cases of this treatment failing? All I see are miraculous healings, but are there cases where B-17 just isn't enough?

Yes. Unfortunately, by the time many patients seek alternative therapies, they have already gone through chemotherapy, radiation, surgery, and there is already extensive damage caused by these orthodox treatments and even the cancer itself. And by the time some people hear about the healing properties of vitamin B-17 it is already too late. B-17 is simply a natural metabolic agent that, under the right circumstances, will help the body get rid of cancer when used as part of a bask nutritional or metabolic therapy which also involves the administration of other vitamins, certain enzymes, and a diet from which animal protein has been mostly removed. It is not to be mistaken for a magic pill that will wipe out cancer and rebuild you a new body.

25) Q. If vitamin B-17 kills cancer-using cyanide, is it possible for the cyanide to kill normal cells?

Absolutely Not. Research shows that the normal cells in our organism contain an enzyme called Rodhanese which "neutralises" the Amygdalin. This enzyme does not allow the Amygdalin to release the cyanide. In this way, Amygdalin only serves as glucose to healthy cells providing energy. Malignant cells do not contain this enzyme. In the absence of Rodhanese, the Amygdalin is activated liberating the cyanide radical only inside the malignant cell causing its destruction (for more information see Laetrile and Cyanide).

26) Q. What do you have to say about articles published on the Internet such as "The Rise and Fall of Laetrile", by Benjamin Wilson, M.D. and Stephen Barrett, M.D. (founder of Quackwatch)?

Several articles have been posted on the Internet to discredit Laetrile making it obvious that one of the two parties involved here is wrong. We have dedicated sections of our web-site to rebut all of these allegations allowing you to be the judge. We would like to invite you to read our section

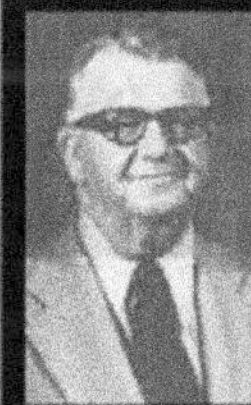

Case Histories

Following are some case histories from my files. The full name is given where permission has been obtained; otherwise, the patient's initials are used.

Polly Todd

This 59-year-old woman was seen by me for the first time on 1/10/75 with the history that she had her left breast removed one month previously because of carcinoma. Three positive nodes had been found. I will let the patient tell you the rest of her history in her own words:

"It was recommended by a prominent physician that I be a part of an experiment in a (then) new chemotherapy program. For a second opinion I went to another city where I had a personal contact with the head of a large hospital. There they told me that my odds of survival were slim, and that I should be treated with strong doses of chemotherapy and radiation. At this point, a friend told me about the Laetrile-nutritional program, which I chose."

The lady was placed on a nutritional program at that time and she has remained on it ever since. She is now 79 years old, in good health, and she has had no recurrence of her disease.

In a recent letter the patient said, "None of the above people on the chemotherapy program lived beyond I 1/2 years. Friends who scoffed at our choice then have much more respect now because others choosing the conventional treatment are gone, while I survive!"

Sue Tarbutton

This 50 year-old woman was seen by me for the first time on 10/26/83 with a history that one week before she had a lump removed from her right breast which was found to be malignant. She did not want to have a mastectomy and wanted to go on a nutritional program.

She has now been on the program for ten years, has had no recurrence of her disease and is quite well.

Elizabeth Winschel

This 51-year-old woman was first seen by me on 10/11/76. Four months before she had been found to have carcinoma of the colon with malignant cells in the abdominal fluid. She had four chemotherapy treatments but discontinued them because they made her so ill. She was started on a nutritional program. Now, seventeen years later, she continues to do well with no recurrence at the primary site of her disease and no metastases.

Wasley Krogdahl

This 60-year-old man was first seen by me on 4/20/79. In November, 1977, he had been diagnosed with having carcinoma of the urinary bladder. The tumor was removed. In February, 1979, three more tumors were removed. He was started on a nutritional program. In April, 1981, and again in November, 1982, some small tumors were removed from his bladder.

He and his wife came to visit me just recently. He is now 75 years old. He has had no further recurrence of his disease. He looks well, says he is feeling well and his wife says, "He is just as hard-headed as ever."

Beverly Batson

This 70-year-old woman was seen by me for the first time on 9/19/88. She had one-half of her stomach removed one month prior because of carcinoma. She received no radiation or chemotherapy. She has been on her nutritional program for five years. Now at the age of 75, she remains well with no recurrence at the primary site or with any metastases.

Jean Henshall

This 48-year-old woman, that I saw for the first time on 9/8/87, had a history of being diagnosed ten months previously with malignant myeloma (a cancer which affects the bone). Her disease affected the bones in the pelvic area. She had received some radiation to that area which relieved the pain. She was started on a nutritional program which pretty much followed the protocol outlined in Chapter Eleven. However, after she had been off of her Laetrile injections for a few months, she was aware that she did not feel as well as she did while on them. She went back on some injections for a few months, and she felt much better. The injections were again stopped, and she remained on the Laetrile pills. This time she noticed no difference. She has now been on the program for six years and is doing well. "I'm doing everything. Even housework is a joy to me because I can do it."

R.H.

This 43-year-old woman was seen by me for the first time on 10/26/79. Two months prior she had been found to have carcinoma of the ovary with metastases throughout the abdomen. She was, at that time, on chemotherapy. We discussed nutritional therapy — what it would do and what it would not do. I saw her next on 11/13/79. She had two chemotherapy treatments by this time, but she had decided to discontinue them and go on a nutritional program.

She stayed on the program until 1982, decided that she was "cured" at that time and went off of the program completely. I saw her on 6/19/84. At this time, she had a tumor running from her right pelvis up into the right upper quadrant of her abdomen. She went back on her nutritional program. I saw her again on 8/1/84. She was feeling very well. The edges of the tumor were much softer and much more difficult to define. When I saw her on 9/2/84, the edges of the tumor were even softer than before.

I did not see her again until 8/20/85. She had been off of her program for 7 or 8 months. Why? It's a long story, and because of "privileged information" I am not free to discuss it. The tumor had enlarged and was now causing abdominal pain and some swelling in the right leg. I put her back on her program, which included some Laetrile injections, and recommended that she have the tumor surgically removed. On 10/1/85, the patient called me to say that she had undergone surgery. She said that the surgeon had found 5 well walled-off tumors that were easily removed. The pathology report, she said, showed mostly "dead" cancer cells.

In 1988 the patient went off her nutritional program. In 1991 she developed a bowel obstruction from her cancer and now has a colostomy. She did go back on her program again and has remained on it. In the three years that have passed since that time, there has been no recurrence of her disease.

Joan Dewiel

This 45-year-old woman first was seen by me on 1/28/80 with a history of having been found to have carcinoma of the colon in September, 1979. Surgery was done, there were no metastases, and she received no radiation or chemotherapy. She was placed on a nutritional program. That was 14 years ago. She is now 59 years old and has had no recurrence of her disease.

Rex Perry

This 42-year-old man that I first saw on 6/27/79 with a history of having malignant lymphoma, which was originally diagnosed in August, 1978. He had 8 months of chemotherapy, which he tolerated very well. His doctors felt, however, that there was a significant amount of disease still present. They wanted to do several more months of chemotherapy and follow this with total body radiation. The patient did not want to do this because of his concern about what it would do to his immune system. He chose, instead, to use the nutritional approach.

It has now been almost 15 years since he started his nutritional therapy. The most satisfying part of such a case history is that this patient has had no further problem with his disease. He is well and very active.

Pauline Wilcox

This 58-year-old woman was seen by me for the first time on 6/14/85 with a history of having had her left breast removed because of carcinoma in 1983. She received no radiation or chemotherapy.

She was placed on a nutritional program at that time. Since she had already gone for two years without any problem, I used only the Laetrile tablets as that part of her nutritional program. She did well on that program until 1988, when she went off of her diet and was taking her vitamins, enzymes and Laetrile only now and then. In November, 1988, she developed a small lesion on her chest wall. This was removed and found to be a spread of her cancer. She went back on her nutritional program again, except this time I added a series of intravenous Laetrile injections. Since then she has had two other small lesions removed from her chest wall which contained some cancer cells. Most importantly, chest x-rays and bone scans done on both occasions were normal. She remains in good health today. As this patient said to me recently, "My doctor is amazed."

Connie Stork

This 24-year-old woman first was seen by me on 2/26/75. Her history was that in 1970 she had been found to have a malignant tumor of the brain. The tumor was partially removed. This was followed by 25 radiation treatments. In October, 1974, another large mass of tumor was removed, but much of the tumor remained. She was told that she had all of the radiation she could have. She was started on a nutritional program.

Now, some 19 years later, Connie has had no recurrence of her tumor. She did have greatly impaired vision as the result of her tumors in 1970 and 1974, and this has progressed to blindness. However, she is still very much alive and is blessed with a healthy mind and healthy body.

Irene Dirks

This 59-year-old woman was seen for the first time on 8/19/80. Her history was that six weeks before I saw her she had been found to have a very low hemoglobin (anemia). She was given blood. Her workup showed that she had a gastric ulcer, but it was questionable whether she had any bleeding from that ulcer. I discussed with her at that time a nutritional program that included some changes in her diet, some vitamins and a small amount of Laetrile by mouth. These changes were obviously not sufficient, because in March, 1981, she began having occasional vaginal bleeding. Two months later this bleeding was found to come from endometrial carcinoma (cancer of the lining of the uterus). A hysterectomy was done, and she was put on the full nutritional program. Now, some 14 years later, she has had no recurrence of her disease and at the age of 73 is quite well and very active.

Doris Dickson

This 50-year-old woman was first seen on 5/14/85 with a history of having had a node removed from the left side of her neck in 1979. From this a diagnosis of lymphatic leukemia was made. She had one chemotherapy treatment, but this made her so ill she discontinued it. She went on a nutritional program of her own, which she stayed on until six months prior to the time I first saw her. She stated that for the past two or three months she had not felt well and that a recent blood count showed a 21,000 white cell count. A white cell count done on the day I saw her was 24,000. (A normal count is about 5,000 to 10,500.)

Mrs. Dickson was started on my nutritional program. I did not feel in her case that the intravenous Laetrile was necessary, so I used just the Laetrile tablets as that part of her program. One month later Mrs. Dickson reported that she was feeling much better. Her white cell count was down to 17,300. Her white cell count continued to drop and by November, 1985, it was down to 9,700.

In June, 1991, Mrs. Dickson reported a gradual increase in fatigue. Her white-cell count was 13,700. I reviewed her nutritional program and found some slips here-and-there that needed to be corrected. By October of that year her cell count was down to 10,700. In a recent letter from her, Mrs. Dickson reports that she is doing well.

T.P.

This 59-year-old man that was seen for the first time on 7/18/80. His history was that one month prior to this a routine x-ray showed a mass in his right lung. A biopsy showed this to be carcinoma. Five radiation treatments were given followed by one chemotherapy treatment that made him so ill he discontinued that whole program. He was started on my nutritional program.

An x-ray done in January, 1981, showed that the tumor in his right lung was completely gone. Let me quote from a letter I received from him on January 23, 1981:

"They were surprised here at [hospital name omitted] comparing the x-ray of last June and the one I just received .... Hope you understand what I am trying to say. I was really tickled when I learned the tumor was gone, and I thought of you right away. I know in my heart it was the Amygdalin and will never think differently.

"The doctor I had at the hospital in June said it was probably the 5 radiation treatments I had. They just don't want to admit [it was the Amygdalin], I guess."

My last contact with this patient was in April, 1993. At that time he was doing very well.

Helyne Victor

This 54-year-old woman was first seen on 6/7/74. In 1967 she had her right breast removed because of cancer. In 1970 she had her left breast removed, also because of cancer. She had received no radiation or chemotherapy after either surgery. While yearly check-ups had failed to find any spread of her disease, this woman just didn't feel well and wanted to get on a good nutritional program.

Mrs. Victor tells her story best. This is from a letter she wrote to the Ohio State Medical Board on April 5, 1975:

"My health has not been good and it was approximately a year ago that I found myself going downhill as far as my health was concerned, not knowing what to do or to whom to go for help. My husband and I began to read and research various avenues for nutritional help or aid.

"I felt very strongly that my poor health may have been due partly to faulty nutrition. After reading materials on proper diets. etc.. I heard of Dr. Binzel and had heard that he did treat patients with a nutritional program. So, I called him and made an appointment ....

"Following a good diet, as he suggested, and taking multiple vitamins for the past year, I can honestly say that I feel like a different person. My health has improved 100%, and I'm feeling like my old self and extremely happy with the results.... "

Mrs. Victor continues to do well. She is now 74 years old and in a recent letter she said of herself and her husband, "We enjoy life and travel a lot."

M.S.

This 62-year-old woman was first seen on 12/6/78. One month previously she had a mole removed from her back. This mole turned out to be a malignant melanoma. She had no radiation or chemotherapy.

She was placed on a nutritional program. She is now 77 years old, quite well and quite active. She has had small a skin cancer removed from her face, but this was not melanoma and was unrelated to her previous disease.

I bring this case to your attention because melanoma is a highly malignant disease which frequently metastasizes rapidly to the liver. This woman was one of 10 patients that I saw with primary malignant melanoma (it had not spread to any other area). To the best of my knowledge, none of those patients have developed metastatic disease.

B.D.

This 62-year-old woman was seen by me for the first time on 5/22/84. In January, 1980, she had been found to have malignant lymphoma. She received chemotherapy from January, 1980.

through November, 1980. In March, 1982, she developed a small nodule in the back portion of her left neck area and a few months later a larger nodule in the right mandibular angle (jaw). She placed herself on a pretty good nutritional program at that time and the nodules had not progressed at all in size.

I up-graded the nutritional program of this patient by adding Vitamin A and Laetrile to what she was already doing. She was followed closely by her family doctor for the next two years. He could not detect any enlargements of these nodules. I saw her again on 4/30/86. I felt that the nodule in the right mandibular angle was the same size as before but was firmer and more movable. I thought the nodule on the left side of the neck was the same size but much firmer than before. The next time I saw this patient was on 2/18/91. I could not find any nodules at all.

It has now been 10 years since she started on her nutritional program. In a recent letter she said, "I am doing well and leading an active life...I continue to take all of the vitamins that you prescribed and I never miss a dose."

B.W.

This 44-year-old woman was seen for the first time on 2/6/81. She had been found one month prior to have carcinoma of the descending colon with 7 positive lymph nodes. A colostomy was not required. She received no radiation or chemotherapy.

She was started on a nutritional program. Now. some 13 years later, she has had no recurrence of her disease and leads a normal, active life.

What is so unusual about this patient? She had cancer of the colon with metastases. The odds of her surviving 5 years were one in one-thousand. Yet, she lives a normal life with no recurrence of her disease after 13 years.

Alice Silverthorn

This 46-year-old woman was seen by me for the first time on 1/5/76. Her left breast had been removed in 1971 because of carcinoma. This was followed by radiation and chemotherapy.

She had just been told that her disease had now spread to the cervical vertebrae (neck), her left rib cage and the vertebrae in her lower back. Her doctors wanted to give her more chemotherapy, but she did not want it. She wanted to go on a nutritional program.

When she started her nutritional program, she was having much pain. Within a month, the pain began to subside. In April, 1976, she began having more pain in her rib cage and in her lower back. She was put back on her intravenous Laetrile three times weekly for two weeks. The pain again subsided. In August of that year she began to have some pain once more in her rib cage. She was given intravenous Laetrile twice weekly for three weeks. Again the pain subsided. It has now been 18 years since she first started on her program. She is 64 years old and doing very well.

Let me share with you part of a letter I recently received from Mrs. Silverthorn:

"I remember only too well the fear and desperation, yes, and downright helplessness, I felt when the doctors at (hospital name deleted) told me the cancer had metastasized to my bones. It was a sentence of 'death.' I was told I would need to start chemo-treatments immediately. There was even talk of taking the pituitary gland out at some later date. I had already had a radical left breast operation and was treated with mustard gas, cobalt and male hormones. I had enough of torture! ! !

"When a friend told me about your nutritional approach to treating diseases, 1 was ready to try it. Even though we both knew my chances of survival were slim, together, we were willing to take on the challenge of fighting for my life. Now, thank God, you can claim me as one of your survivors.

"I hope you include in your book how we feel, and just how difficult it is for those of us who were supposed to die, when the medical profession and well-meaning, intelligent people make the suggestion that the only reason we are alive is because it was a mis-diagnosis or the disease has gone into a 'spontaneous' remission. Most people make us feel like psychiatric patients. It is difficult to explain miracles, yet, that is what happened."

Grace Laman

This 59-year-old woman was seen for the first time on 10/5/76. She had been diagnosed as having carcinoma of the pancreas six months prior to this. The only thing that had been done surgically was to run a tube from her bile duct to the outside. She was on chemotherapy for two months but stopped it herself because it made her so ill. She was told at that time that she had only 6 months to live. She was placed on a nutritional program.

Let me quote part of a letter I received from her almost two years later (9/23/78):

"I was [recently] put through a new scanner which showed that my tumor had reduced to the size of a tennis ball. It had been the size of [the doctor's] hand, so he said."

Now, 18 years later, she is 77 years old. In the letter which accompanied her picture she said, "This is my activity picture of me eating out, which I do very well."

Note: With surgery and/or radiation and/or chemotherapy the chances of surviving more than one year with cancer of the pancreas are about I in 10,000.

E.D.

This 57-year-old man was first seen on 4/28/92 (and for that reason is not included in my statistical study) with a history of a diagnosis of carcinoma of the left lung 10 months previously. Surgery had been done followed by one chemotherapy treatment. This made him so ill that he discontinued it. He was then given 25 radiation treatments ending in December, 1991. In March, 1992, x-rays showed extensive growth of the tumors in that lung. He was placed on a nutritional program.

X-rays done in July, 1993, showed no further growth of the tumors in the left lung. X-rays done in November, 1993, showed that the tumors had all become scar tissue. In the most recent letter I received from him he stated that he was feeling so well that "I have no right to complain, so I have to cuss a lot about taxes, politicians, etc." (Alive And Well)

"Laetrile is another key component for keeping cancer from growing and should be considered a standard, entirely safe treatment for all cancer patients." by Dr. Atkins., M.D.

~~**~~

After more than twenty years of such specialized work, I have found the non-toxic Laetrile is far superior to any other known cancer treatment. In my opinion it is the only existing possibility for the ultimate control of cancer. by Dr. Nieper (from the book "World Without Cancer by Edward Griffin")

~~**~~

Laetrile can control cancer. But it is not widely available to the public, because it cannot be patented, and therefore is not commercially attractive to the pharmaceutical industry. – "The Science and Politics of Cancer" by G. Edward Griffin

~~**~~

I have been using Laetrile in the treatment of cancer since the mid1970s and our success is astounding. He tells of his ongoing battle with the medical establishment, but this is primarily the story of his alive-and-well patients. by Dr. Philip E. Binzel, Jr., M.D.

~~**~~

So, here is a bureau of the Federal Government which, a short time before, had said that the reason Laetrile did not work was because it did not release hydrogen cyanide in the presence of cancer cells. Now, when they find that it does, they say that it is toxic. When offered an opportunity to present evidence of Laetrile's toxicity in Federal Court, they admitted that they had none. From Laetrile and the Life Saving Substance Called Cyanide by Philip Binzel, Jr., M.D.

~~**~~

Certainly one story that needs to be told is that of Dr. Kanematsu Sugiura. In 1975, Dr. Sugiura was, and had been for some years, one of the most respected cancer research scientists at Sloan-Kettering. In working with cancerous mice, Dr. Sugiura found that, when he used Laetrile on these mice, seventy-seven per cent of them did not develop a spread of their disease (metastatic carcinoma). He repeated this study over and over for two years. The results were always the same. Dr. Sugiura took his findings to his superiors at Sloan-Kettering, but his study was never published. Instead, Sloan-Kettering published the results of someone else who claimed that he had used Dr. Sugiura's protocol. This "someone else's" study showed that there were no beneficial effects from the use of Laetrile. Dr. Sugiura complained. He was fired. A book was written about all of this entitled The Anatomy of A Cover-up. This book has all the actual results of Dr. Sugiura's work. These results do, indeed, show the benefit of Laetrile. Dr. Sugiura stated in this book, "It is still my belief that Amygdalin cures metastases." Amygdalin is, of course, the scientific name for Laetrile. ALIVE AND WELL by Philip E. Binzel, Jr., M.D.

~~**~~

I ... have specialized in oncology [the study of tumors] for the past eighteen years. For the same number of years I have been using Laetrile—amygdalin in the treatment of my cancer patients. During this eighteen year period I have treated a total of over five hundred patients with Laetrile—amygdalin by various routes of administration, including the oral and the I.V. The majority of my patients receiving Laetrile—amygdalin have been in a terminal state when treatment with this material commenced. It is my carefully considered clinical judgment, as a practicing oncologist and researcher in this field, that I have obtained most significant and encouraging results with the use of Laetrile—amygdalin in the treatment of terminal cancer patients, and that these results are comparable or superior to the results I have obtained with the use of the more toxic standard cytotoxic agents. By Navarro, M.D., Manuel

"Laetrile is most assuredly a very potent anti-cancer factor but requires stringent methods of use in order to succeed. Amateurs invariably fail. High sounding U.S. pronouncements that 'laetrile' is toxic and ineffective are fraudulent and calculated to deceive. It will become again one of the major weapons in the cancer therapy armamentarium." By Dr Richards & Frank Hourigan.

"You get cats in with high fevers, 105-108 degrees. There is nothing you can give them that will bring down that high a fever--except laetrile."---Dr Kearns, DVM. (Dr Kearns uses 50mg of laetrile orally until the leukemia is under control.)

Administered to cancer patients, Laetrile has proven to be quite free from any harmful side-effects, and I would say that no anti-cancer drug could make a cancerous patient improve faster than Laetrile. It goes without saying that Laetrile controls cancer and is quite effective wherever it is located. By Shigeaki Sakai, a prominent physician in Tokyo. [World Without Cancer by Edward Griffin]

In Italy there is Professor Etore Guidetti, M.D., of the University of Turin Medical School. Dr. Guidetti spoke before the Conference of the International Union Against Cancer held in Brazil in 1954 and revealed how his use of Laetrile in terminal cancer patients had caused the destruction of a wide variety of tumors including those of the uterus, cervix, rectum, and breast. "In some cases," he said, "one has been able to observe a group of fulminating and cauliflower-like neoplastic masses resolved very rapidly" He reported that, after giving Laetrile to patients with lung cancer, he had been "able to observe, with the aid of radiography, a regression of the neoplasm or the metastases." [World Without Cancer by Edward Griffin]

~~**~~

"The cyano group of vitamin B-12 (cyano-cobal-amin) is more labile and potentially more harmful than the cyano group found in Laetrile. Yet we know how safe and essential vitamin B-12 is." - Dr. R.A. Passwater, testimony, FDA docket # 77N-0048.

~~**~~

"When Dr. Manner reported on the total remission of breast cancer in lab animals (Using 'Laetrile in conjunction with vitamins and enzymes'), ACS President, Ben Byrd, criticized (him) for making his announcement in public, and said such announcements should be made only in a proper scientific forum."

~~**~~

(Laetrile)" may be useful in sickle cell anemia...(Laetrile) used in animals with tumors show: a decrease in lung metastases; slower tumor growth; and pain relief." - Lloyd Old, MD, vice president, Sloan-Kettering Institute for Cancer Research, at FDA 7-2-1974.

~~**~~

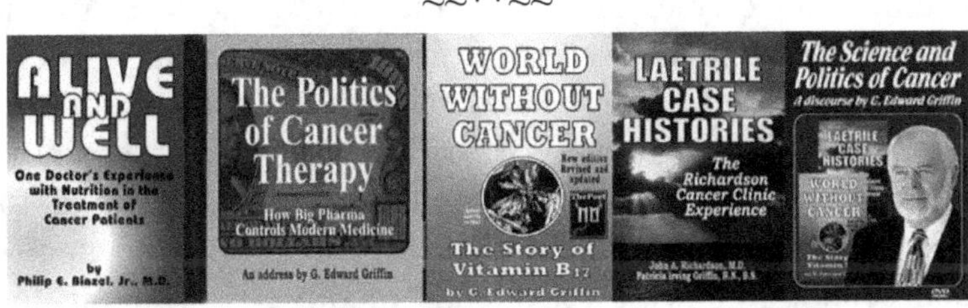

Dr. Philip E. Binzel – "Alive And Well"

Dr. Philip E. Binzel, a native of Bowling Green, Kentucky, was a graduate of the Medical School at St. Louis University in Missouri and did his internship at Christ Hospital in Cincinnati, Ohio. In 1955 he entered Family Practice in Washington Court House, Ohio.

In 1974, he began to investigate the role of nutrition in human disorders and came to the conclusion that this was an important field of knowledge. Cautiously, he began to incorporate that knowledge into his medical practice and, based on personal experience, developed a highly effective protocol for the treatment of a wide range of disorders, including cancer.

Dr. Binzel started using Laetrile and other nutritional therapies in the treatment of cancer patients since the mid 1970s. His record of success is astounding. Medical case histories of his patients are included in this book. G. Edward Griffin encouraged and persuaded him to write a book on Laetrile and so he wrote the great book "Alive And Well".

Mr. Edward Griffin: The Story of Vitamin B-17

Mr. G. Edward Griffin marshals the evidence that cancer is a deficiency disease - like scurvy or pellagra - aggravated by the lack of an essential food compound in modern man s diet. That substance is vitamin B17. In its purified form developed for cancer therapy, it is known as Laetrile. This story is not approved by orthodox medicine. The FDA, the AMA, and The American Cancer Society have labeled it fraud and quackery. Yet the evidence is clear that here, at last, is the final answer to the cancer riddle. Why has orthodox medicine waged war against this non drug approach? The author contends that the answer is to be found, not in science, but in politics - and is based upon the hidden economic and power agenda of those who dominate the medical establishment. This is the most complete and authoritative treatise available on this topic.

Dr. Ernesto Contreras: Oasis of Hope

In 1963, the late Dr. Ernsto Contreras, Sr. opened the Oasis of Hope Hospital and initiated what would become a healing tradition known as the Total Cancer Care Approach. Dr. Contreras is recognized in multiple publications as a pioneer in body, mind, and spirit medicine. At the foundation of his philosophy were two principles inspired by Hippocrates, the father of medicine, and Jesus Christ, The Great Physician: 1) First, do no harm; 2) Love your patient as you love yourself.

Because of his philosophy, Dr. Contreras taught his medical staff to never prescribe treatments that would destroy the quality of life of the patient. He also insisted that Oasis of Hope physicians offer therapies that they would be willing to take if in the same circumstances. His emphasis on the doctor-patient relationship, along with his integration of natural and conventional therapies with emotional and spiritual counseling, were the 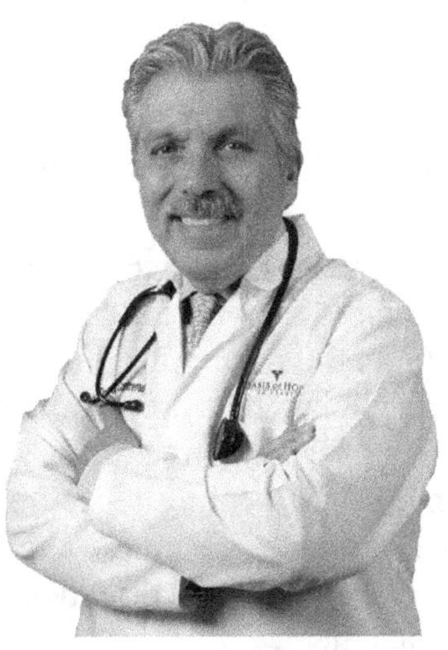 principle reasons why more than 100,000 patients from 55 nations have come to Oasis of Hope for treatment over the last 45 years.

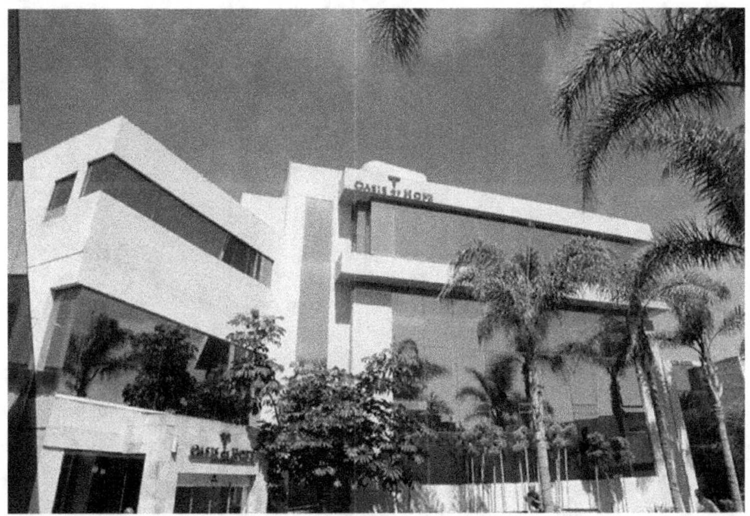

Dr. Contreras believed that to be effective as a physician, one had to blend art and science. When treating cancer patients,

Dr. Contreras looked beyond the obvious. He would find the root needs of his patients and develop personalized therapies to address the unique circumstance of each. His commitment to treat his patients with professionalism, ethics, and compassion made him a beloved doctor. As a researcher, Dr. Contreras explored hundreds of treatment modalities in his constant quest to help his patients. His untiring determination inspired his staff and patients alike.

At age 88, after 62 years of medical practice, Dr. Contreras went on to be with the Lord. Two of his significant contributions to humanity were his model for integrative medicine and the development of a tremendous platform for the advancement of cancer research, treatment, and control. The Oasis of Hope is home of the healing legacy of Dr. Ernsto Contreras, Sr. and the staff continues to utilize the Total Care Approach and develop and design new and effective protocols for comprehensive cancer management.

Address: OASIS of Hope Hospital in Fracc. Playas de Tijuana, Terrazas, 22504 Tijuana, Baja California, Mexico, you may visit them on the web at http://www.oasisofhope.com or Phone +52 664 631 6100

Disclaimer

This book is not intended to replace the advice and/or care of a qualified health care professional. Please do not try to self diagnose or self treat any disease. Seek professional help and consult your physician before making any dietary changes.

This book is not intended to provide medical advice and is sold with the understanding that the publisher and the author have neither liability nor responsibility to any person or entity with respect to loss, damage or injury caused or alleged to be caused directly or indirectly by the information contained in this book or the use of any products mentioned. Readers should not use any of the product discussed in this book without the advice of a medical professional.

The Food and Drug Administration has not approved the use of any of the natural treatments discussed in this book. This book, and the information contained herein, has not been approved by the Food and the Drug Administration.

Cancer - Cause and Cure: Based on Quantum Physics developed by Dr. Johanna Budwig

http://www.amazon.com/Cancer-Quantum-Physics-developed-Johanna-ebook/dp/B00P3Y7BYG

Book Description

***** A must have book for every cancer patient *****

This book provides an introduction of Dr. Budwig's cancer research and treatment. Johanna Budwig (1908-2003) was nominated for the Nobel Prize seven times. She was one of Germany's leading scientists of the 20th Century, a biochemist and cancer specialist with a special interest in essential fats.

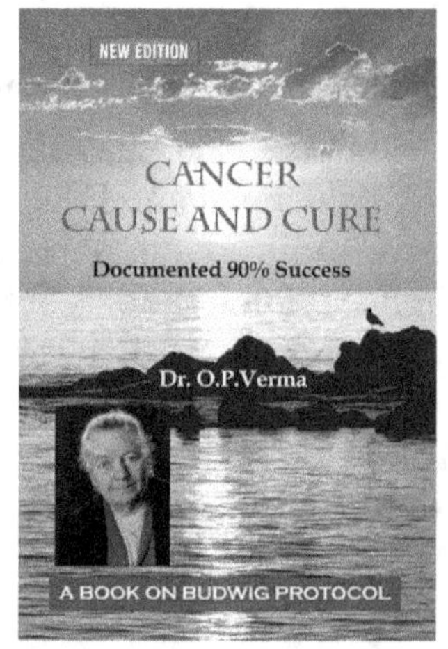

Otto Warburg proved that prime cause of cancer oxygen-deficiency in the cells. In absence of oxygen cells ferment glucose to produce energy, lactic acid is formed as a byproduct of fermentation. He postulated that sulfur containing protein and some unknown fat is required to attract oxygen in the cell.

In 1951 Dr. Budwig developed Paper Chromatography to identify fats. With this technique she proved that electron rich highly unsaturated Linoleic and Linolenic fatty acids were the undiscovered mysterious decisive fats in respiratory enzyme function that Otto Warburg had been unable to find. She studied the electromagnetic function of pi-electrons of the linolenic acid in the membranes of the microstructure of protoplasm, for all nerve function, secretions, mitosis, as well as cell break-down. This immediately caused lot of excitement in the scientific community. New doors could open in Cancer research. Hydrogenated fats, including all Trans fatty acids were proved as respiratory poisons.

Then Budwig decided to have human trials and gave flaxseed oil and quark to cancer patients. After three months, the patients began to improve in health and strength, the yellow green substance in their blood began to disappear, tumors gradually receded and at the same time the nutrients began to rise. This way Dr. Budwig had found a cure for cancer. It was a great victory and first milestone in the battle against cancer. Her treatment protocol is based on the consumption of flax seed oil with low fat cottage cheese, raw organic diet, mild exercise, and the healing powers of the sun. She treated approx. 2500 cancer patients during a 50 year period with this protocol till her death with over 90% documented success.

She was nominated 7 times for Nobel Prize but with a condition that she will use chemotherapy and radiotherapy with her protocol. They did not want to collapse the 200 billion dollar business over night. She always refused to support the damaging chemo and radio for the sake of humanity.

Lothar Hirneise is founder and President of People Against Cancer, Germany. He travels a lot in search of finding most successful alternative cancer therapies. He has been student of Dr. Johanna Budwig. He is a great researcher and writer on alternative healing. He is successfully treating thousands of cancer patients at his 3-E center in Germany. In the last few years he has interviewed several hundred final stage so-called survivors, meaning patients who were in the final stage of cancer and who are all healthy again today. Based on his findings he proposed a 3 E Program – The Mnemonic of Cancer Treatment.

   1) Eat well

   2) Eliminate

   3) Energy

He noticed that 100% of all survivors, did the energy work. In approximately - say 80% of all patients, had changed their diet. And in at least 60% of all patients, took intensive detoxification rituals. This is the basis of his, so much talked about 3E Program for healing cancer.

Lothar Hirneise strongly supports holistic and spiritual approach and includes Visualization, Tumor Contract, Meditation, mild Yoga, Emotional Freedom Technique, Dr. Ryke Geerd Hamer's New German Medicine (Connection of unresolved stress and cancer), Detoxification techniques (Soda Bicarb bath, Epsom bath, Sauna, Colon Hydrotherapy, Coffee Enema etc.) in his 3 E Program.

The book also, describes about rare and miraculous herbs used in the treatment of Cancer like Turmeric, Black seed, Ginger, Mistle Toe, Aloe vera, Echinecea, Lobelia, Essiac Tea, Pau d'arco Tea, Dandelion, Milk Thistle.

~~**~~

Available on Amazon.com

Awesome Flax: A Book by Flax Guru

Flax seed- Miraculous Anti-ageing Divine Food

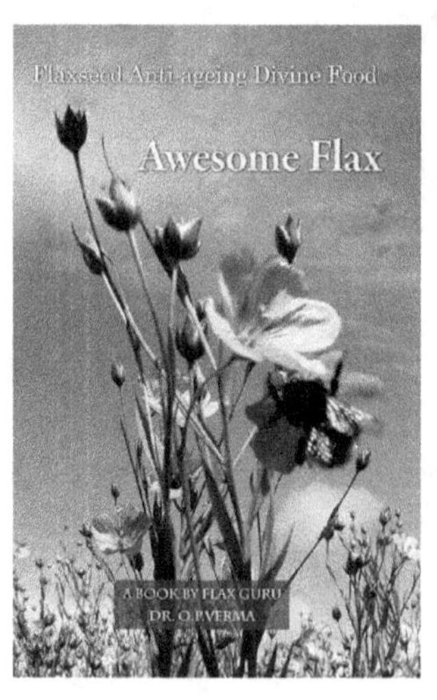

What is Flax seed and how can it benefit me? I was faced with this question when I started hearing about Flax seed not long ago. It became a 'buzz word' in society and seems to be making great role in increased health for many. I wanted to join that wagon of wellness and so I researched until I felt satisfied that it could help me, too. Here are my findings.

Flax seeds are the hard, tiny seeds of Linum usitatissimum, the Flax plant, which has been widely used for thousands of years as a source of food and clothing. Flax seeds have become very popular recently, because they are a richest source of the Omega 3 essential fatty acid; also known as Alpha Linolenic Acid (ALA) and lignans. People in the new millennium may see Flax seed as an important new FOOD SUPER STAR. In fact, there's nobody who won't benefit by adding Flax seed to his or her diet. Even Gandhi wrote: "Wherever Flax seed becomes a regular food item among the people, there will be better health."

Flax seed contains 30-40% oil (including 36-50% alpha linolenic acid, 23-24% linoleic acid- Omega-6 fatty acids and oleic acids), mucilage (6%), protein (25%), Vitamin B group, lecithin, selenium, calcium, folate, magnesium, zinc, iron, carotene, sulfur, potassium, phosphorous, manganese, silicon, copper, nickel, molybdenum, chromium, and cobalt, vitamins A and E and all essential amino acids.

Other fatty acids, omega-6's, is abundant in vegetable oils such as corn, soybean, safflower, and sunflower oils as well as in the many processed foods made from these oils. Omega-6 fatty acids have stimulating, irritating and inflammatory effect while omega-3 fatty acids have calming and soothing effect on our body. Our bodies function best when our diets contain a well-balanced ratio of these fatty acids, meaning 1:1 to 4:1 of omega-6 and omega-3. But we typically eat 10 to 30 times more omega-6 than omega-3's, which is a prescription for trouble. This imbalance puts us at greater risk for a number of serious illnesses, including heart disease, cancer, stroke, and arthritis. As the most abundant plant source of omega-3 fatty acids, Flax seed helps restore balance and lets omega-3's do what they're best at: balancing the immune system, decreasing inflammation, and lowering some of the risk factors for heart disease.

One way that Omega 3 essential fatty acid known as Alpha Linolenic Acid ALA helps the heart is by decreasing the ability of platelets to clump together. Flax seed helps to lower high blood pressure, clears clogged coronaries, lowers high blood cholesterol, bad LDL cholesterol and triglyceride levels and raises good HDL cholesterol. It can relieve the symptoms of

Diabetes Mellitus. It lowers blood sugar level. Flax seed help fight obesity. Adding Flax seed to foods creates a feeling of satiation. Furthermore, Flax seed stokes the metabolic processes in our cells. Much like a furnace, once stoked, the cells generate more heat and burn calories.

Flax seeds are the most abundant source of lignans. Lignans are plant-based compounds that can block estrogen activity in cells, reducing the risk of Breast, Uterus, Colon and Prostate cancers. According to the US Department of Agriculture, Flax seed contains 27 identifiable cancer preventative compounds. Lignans in Flax seeds are 200 to 800 times more than any other lignan source. Lignans are phytoestrogens, meaning that they are similar to but weaker than the estrogen that a woman's body produces naturally. Therefore, they may also help alleviate menopausal discomforts such as hot flashes and vaginal dryness. They are also antibacterial, antifungal, and antiviral.

Because they are high in dietary fiber, ground Flax seeds can help ease the passage of stools and thus relieve constipation, hemorrhoids and diverticular disease. Taken for inflammatory bowel disease, Flax seed can help to calm inflammation and repair any intestinal tract damage.

Secrets of Success: Smart way to success for every student

Secrets of Success

Normally people think that memory, intelligence or learning ability is a God gift and it is not possible to further improve or increase the brain powers. We take it for granted that it will remain as it is gifted to us by God. But the truth is just opposite. Understand that as you go to gym for workout to develop your six pack abs, feed your body with muscle building food and get sharp sculpted body shape. Friends, believe me if muscle can be built and remodeled, then why not your brain's hardware and circuit boards. If you feed your brain with proper food it needs, follow simple instructions and take advantage of neurobics or mnemonics, you can immensely increase your brain's abilities.

We have tremendous powers locked inside our brains, but we are not using them to full extent. Dr. William James, considered the father of modern psychology, pointed out that "the average human being uses only 10 percent of his mental capacity." We still have to find out how much power or secrets are hidden in our brain.

Nowadays scientists have discovered mysterious techniques and nutrients to boost our brain powers. Today I shall raise curtains from all these secrets; I shall disclose all hidden tricks and tips. Today you are going to learn how your CPU, the brain tightly packed in a bony cabinet, functions. I teach you how each component and microprocessors works and how the best insulation material can be prepared. I also disclose the right technique to sharpen your brain and to make you an intelligent and successful scholar.

Today you will learn how to crack every examination you face, solve every question, defeat every opponent and get highest possible marks. You are going to write new equation of education and success.

Friends new boundaries and horizon of success is ready to welcome you. Today we shall discuss in detail about some great nutrients and supplements to boost your memory, learning, imagination, creativity and concentration. If you follow our suggestions and apply simple tricks you achieve a successful personality. This short e-book is going to prove a turning point in your life. Wish you luck.

www.ingramcontent.com/pod-product-compliance
Lightning Source LLC
Chambersburg PA
CBHW071229240726
48654CB00009B/970